Praise for

The Tenth Nerve

"[Honey is] a caring and compassionate physician and an impressive prose stylist. Writing well for a general audience about the complexities of the brain and the challenges of neurosurgery can be a daunting task. . . . Honey takes on the challenge in this compelling human document and tells his stories in polished, engaging prose that moves smoothly from vivid descriptions of brain surgery to profiles of his patients and colleagues, to good-humoured wit, often at his own expense. . . . If *The Tenth Nerve* confined itself to a mere display of the author's impressive erudition and clinical experience it would be a perfectly adequate addition to the world of popular science, but it would be a lesser book than the one that Honey has crafted here. . . . This is a terrific book. Highly recommended." —*Vancouver Sun*

"In this revealing memoir, Chris Honey weaves impressive surgical knowledge and thrilling medical history together with real patient cases, allowing the reader to bear witness to a modern-day medical breakthrough. Beautifully written and accessible, *The Tenth Nerve* features the touching stories of patients who profoundly impacted Dr. Honey's career and transformed him personally." —Dr. Christian Smith, author of *The Scientist and the Psychic: A Son's Exploration of His Mother's Gift*

"In *The Tenth Nerve*, Chris Honey shows us more than the neurosurgeon's hidden world—the chaos of the emergency, the ache of the hopeless patient, the subtly pulsing moonscape of the brain under an operating microscope. His is a heartfelt and informed story about crafting a working wisdom, an acumen, about his patients, his profession and, ultimately, himself." —Dr. Liam Durcan, author of *The Measure of Darkness* and *Garcia's Heart*

"A new book by the Head of Neurosurgery [at the University of British Columbia] offers a fresh perspective about medicine and a riveting look into neurosurgical operating rooms. . . . Honey's new book brings the reader into the operating room and reveals the impact that patient and surgeon have on each other's lives." —*The Ubyssey*

The
Tenth Nerve

A Brain Surgeon's Stories
of the Patients Who Changed Him

Chris Honey, MD

Vintage Canada

Published by Vintage Canada, a division of Penguin Random House Canada
Limited, Toronto, 2023. Previously published in hardcover in Canada by Random
House Canada, a division of Penguin Random House Canada Limited, Toronto,
2021. Distributed by Penguin Random House Canada Limited, Toronto.

Vintage Canada and colophon are registered trademarks.

www.penguinrandomhouse.ca

The author has changed the names of some of the individuals in this book,
and in some cases modified identifying details in order to preserve anonymity.

Library and Archives Canada Cataloguing in Publication
Title: The tenth nerve : a brain surgeon's stories of the patients
who changed him / Christopher Honey.
Names: Honey, Christopher, author.
Identifiers: Canadiana 20210256478 | ISBN 9781039001183 (softcover)
Subjects: LCSH: Honey, Christopher. | LCSH: Neurosurgeons—Canada—
Biography. | LCSH: Nervous system—Surgery—Patients—Anecdotes. |
LCSH: Nervous system—Surgery—Anecdotes. | LCGFT: Autobiographies.
Classification: LCC RD592.9.H66 A3 2023 | DDC 617.4/8092—dc23

Cover design: Dylan Browne
Cover image: (texture) Pakin Songmor / Getty Images;
(brain) Mirror-images / Adobe Stock Images
Interior design: Andrew Roberts

Printed in the United States of America

2 4 6 8 9 7 5 3 1

Penguin
Random House
VINTAGE CANADA

To Karla with love

CONTENTS

Foreword

For most people, neurosurgery is a mysterious, high-stakes profession—that's part of the reason I was drawn to it as a curious child and, eventually, as a medical intern and doctoral student. Even after centuries of medical exploration, the brain, lying hidden and protected beneath the skull, is rarely seen and only superficially understood. It is the precious organ responsible for our thoughts, movements and personality—to operate on the brain invites the danger of changing the very essence of the patient. Not a casual endeavour.

After practising neurosurgery for more than twenty-five years, I wrote this book to show how a brain surgeon operates—literally—and to share the human stories behind two significant discoveries by my team at Vancouver General Hospital of previously unrecognized but likely ancient diseases. In recounting these events, I realized that some of my patients had profoundly changed who I was.

Here, then, is a book about discoveries—both medical discoveries that I have provided my patients and personal discoveries that my patients have prompted in me. These are the stories of seven brave individuals whose close encounters changed me into a better person and surgeon. The scalpel can only go so deep, and technical skill can only take you so far. Real understanding of an illness requires listening and genuine care. *The Tenth Nerve* is a book about curiosity, the wonder of the human brain, and the courage of a few remarkable patients.

In the 1500s, when medical knowledge and treatments were limited, doctors provided more emotional support than medical cure. The French surgeon Ambroise Paré (1510–1590) famously said, "The physician's duty is to cure occasionally, relieve often, console always." Nowadays, these duties have been reversed in importance. Doctors are expected to cure always and leave the consoling to the nurses.

On the first day of medical school, the cadavers have their faces and hands wrapped in white linen to limit any emotional engagement for the would-be physicians. This practice enhances the ability of the students to dispassionately cut into the bodies and learn their anatomy. By graduation four years later, every student knows doctors should never become emotionally connected to their patients.

We diagnose, we treat, we leave.

If you are foolish enough to become emotionally involved with your patients, they will take you to euphoric highs and suicidal lows. Every day, a doctor kills themself in the United States. In Canada, suicide is the only cause of mortality that is higher among physicians than the general public. Many factors may explain this epidemic of medical suicide, but a key one is the emotional strain of sharing a patient's fears, frustrations and failures. Simply put, riding a roller coaster of compassion entails a very real personal risk to the physician.

The current model of medicine therefore encourages a personal detachment between doctor and patient. That dispassionate approach, coupled with the time pressures of the business of medicine, often leaves the patient feeling that they are just a disease and not a person. The truth, of course, is that the disease and the patient cannot be separated. As Sir William Osler said, "The good physician treats the disease; the great physician treats the patient who has the disease." The superb family doctor knows this, and every medical decision they make is framed by how it will affect the patient and their family.

The virtuoso surgeon, however, need only know how to get that last piece of tumour off the blood vessel without tearing it. Surgeons are expected to be bold, confident and technically gifted. Sometimes wrong but never in doubt. In our weekly neurosurgical morbidity and mortality rounds, cases are discussed in an effort to prevent medical errors from reoccurring. The chief resident begins, "This forty-nine-year-old brain tumour had a craniotomy with gross total resection last Monday and a few days later developed seizures . . ." The fact that the patient's wife thought he would die and will always remember him shaking uncontrollably is of no relevance. We discuss only why the nameless, forty-nine-year-old "brain tumour" developed his seizures and whether we could have prevented it.

Emotions, we are taught, are an impediment to the best practice of surgery.

But despite all our training to be detached and rational, sometimes a patient does leave an indelible mark on your soul. That is why my first story is about an infant named Saika whom I operated on in Tappita, Liberia, someone who completely changed how I practised medicine and how I viewed the world. I now realize that despite my learned dispassionate approach, a few patients have profoundly changed my understanding of both medicine and myself. In short, they have expanded my understanding of what it means to be human.

1.

SAIKA

I touched down at Roberts International Airport on the outskirts of Monrovia, the capital city of Liberia in West Africa, in the late evening of March 31, 2014, as part of an international aid mission that would perform the first neurosurgical operations in that country.

The team supporting this effort was the Korle-Bu Neuroscience Foundation. A group of nurses and physicians, initially from Vancouver General Hospital, had helped set up and equip a neurosurgery service in neighbouring Ghana. The director of that foundation, Marj Ratel, learned that Liberia had never had a neurosurgeon and wanted to set up a satellite clinic. I had been to Ghana on several occasions to help their neurosurgeons, so she asked if I would come along and help in Liberia.

Our plan was to identify a local general surgeon who was interested in the field and help train them to provide this care for Liberians. We knew that to fly in, operate on a few patients, and then leave without training someone to carry on the work would be a futile drop in the bucket. We needed local buy-in.

Inquiries to the Liberian government revealed that the deputy minister of health, Dr. Francis Kateh, happened to run a hospital with the only CT (computerized tomography) scanner in the country. The Jackson F. Doe Memorial Regional Referral Hospital was located in Tappita, about a six-hour drive east of Monrovia. This hospital had been built by the People's Republic of China. It was inaugurated on February 7, 2011, as a gift from the country and came fully stocked with a variety of diagnostic machines. Around the same time, the China-Union Mining Company secured a twenty-five-year iron ore mining agreement from the Liberian prime minister, the Nobel laureate Ms. Ellen Johnson Sirleaf.

In anticipation of our mission, the foundation had sent an African neurosurgeon from Nigeria to the Jackson F. Doe hospital a month earlier to see patients and identify some for potential surgery. He saw more than two hundred people; at least a dozen were now waiting for their neurosurgery if conditions were right for me to proceed. This would be their only chance for the surgery they needed—without treatment, most would suffer paralysis and succumb to a shortened, painful life. While I was flying across the Atlantic, these prospective patients were living in large open-air ward rooms with their families, who were cooking and cleaning for them.

I spent the first night in a hotel room in Monrovia while we waited for transportation to the hospital on the other side of the country. Monrovia is named after the fifth American president, James Monroe, who had supported a policy of migration of free African Americans to the continent of Africa in the 1820s. Some 4,500 emigrated (or were forced to emigrate by slave owners afraid of the concept of free people of colour and by white supremacists who could not imagine sharing a society with them) to what would become Liberia. More than 60 percent of the migrants died on the journey.

The next morning, I toured the city and gave a lecture at the John F. Kennedy Medical Center. The streets were packed with a mix of car horns, pungent smells and riotous colour. Donkey carts full of vegetables manoeuvred around double-parked cars, while bicycles overladen with the entire day's goods wove in and out. A chaotic scene, but without the anger similar circumstances would cause back home. Everyone was going about their business, and the horns seemed more *I'm here* than *Get out of my way.*

The foundation had promised a United Nations helicopter to Tappita, but that fell through and the only alternative was a long drive over the red dirt roads. Our driver joked that the road, notorious for breaking car axles and trapping buses in the mud, had killed more people getting to the hospital than the hospital had ever saved.

My wife, Karla, phoned me the evening before our departure and asked if I knew that Ebola had just broken out in the country—she had seen a BBC report about it. I told her I didn't and, feeling some fear, sat down to hear the details. Unbeknownst to me, on the day of my arrival, in the district of Foya, a seven-hour drive north of Monrovia near the border with Guinea and Sierra Leone, a young woman had died of the Ebola virus.

There was no mention of the incident in the local newspapers or on the television, and there would be no mention of Ebola in the Liberian media for a few more days. When the outbreak was finally announced in the *Monrovia Times*, there were two front-page articles side by side. One was from Lewis Brown, the minister of information, cultural affairs, and tourism, saying that there was absolutely no Ebola in Liberia. The other, from Walter Gwenigale, the minister of health and social welfare, saying that there was—and please send money. I admired the editor's decision to juxtapose the statements.

The minister of health was correct. The outbreak in Foya quickly killed twelve people, but then no more fatalities were reported for a week, which prompted the minister of information to mistakenly sound the all-clear. The disease would later spread to Monrovia and trigger panic, mistrust and violence among its citizens. Ultimately, this Ebola epidemic would kill 11,315 people, five times more than all the previous outbreaks since the virus was discovered in 1976.

When I met Dr. Kateh upon my arrival in Tappita and saw that he was setting up what looked like isolation tents near a drainage ditch outside the hospital, I understood that Ebola was an imminent threat. He assured me there was nothing to worry about and that he was arranging these isolation facilities just as a precaution. But the fact that these tents were lined up just above a drainage ditch and not inside the hospital was disconcerting. Were they expecting to be over-whelmed? Dr. Kateh wore thick green rubber gloves up to his elbows and avoided the customary handshake with a polite wave.

Though the news was concerning, I didn't think much about the epidemic while I was in Tappita. There was very little I could do about it, and I was there to focus on neurosurgery patients. I assured myself I was far more likely to get malaria than Ebola.

I walked around the hospital to explore its facilities and relieve the left hip pain the bumpy road trip there had caused. The hospital was a white, square, two-storey structure with a red tile roof and a paved courtyard at its centre. Someone was constantly sweeping the floors of the wards with a straw broom; the windows were large and open to facilitate a breeze. There was air conditioning in the operating rooms and the staff lounge, but not on the wards.

The hot air was humid and scented with vegetation as I circled the outside of the building. My long pants and long-sleeved loose shirt, ideal for malaria defence, were soon soaked through. At the back of the compound was a large locked shed humming with the sounds and smells of a diesel generator providing the hospital with electricity. There were two diesel generators that ran one at a time, twelve hours each. I would later learn that the engineers switched the power source from one to the other at 10 a.m. and 10 p.m., allowing each generator to alternately rest or be repaired as needed.

The Chinese donors had left behind five engineers, who were responsible for fixing everything. They had a two-year tour of duty at the hospital before they could go home, and my local Liberian hosts said the Chinese workers were not pleased with this arrangement. It seemed harsh to me as well. There was nothing to do in Tappita—this was not Kruger National Park or Etosha. There was no local wildlife except for some chickens and a few very angry dogs. The workers spent most of their time sitting in their rooms and, according to my hosts, dreaming up excuses not to fix the equipment. The party line was "the equipment needs a new part." New parts were ordered from China and then shipped by container only once a year.

I walked through the empty courtyard, but with the reflection of the sun off the white stones, the heat was oppressive, so I sought out the air-conditioned room for the staff on the bottom floor of the administrative wing. A quarter of the hospital was reserved for its administration. Just like Vancouver General, there were too many bureaucrats and too few doctors. Some things are universal.

That cooled room became our home base when we were not in the operating room. There was a long wooden boardroom-style table in the middle with a dozen wooden chairs around it, a pull-down screen on the far wall, and an LCD projector on the table ready to connect to a laptop computer. I would use the room for my daily teaching rounds.

We also met there for delicious, locally catered meals three times a day. Chicken and rice were the staples—a leaner and more sinewy chicken than I was used to. There was an abundance of local fruit and vegetables, but I avoided it for fear of a diarrheal illness. Two weeks without greens was unpleasant. Two weeks without a beer was punishing. The hospital had a religious zeal, and I assumed they felt Jesus did not share a beer with his mates after a day of miracles.

The medical staff and our team met in the late afternoon each day for teaching rounds, and then we would discuss all the patients and select who would get surgery the next morning. The candidates were a young man in his early thirties, in a wheelchair, with a brain tumour; two infants with massively enlarged heads; a woman with a skull tumour; and half a dozen older people who could not walk more than a few steps because the severe arthritis in their lower back was crushing the nerves to their legs.

Nothing seemed unduly difficult. Back home we could operate on all these patients in a day or two, but in Tappita, it would take ten—at a rate of one operation a day. When I suggested we should do more than one case a day, a few of the more senior members of the team flashed me knowing smiles.

"This is Africa," someone said. "You'll see."

———

The woman with the skull tumour had been operated on the day before I arrived by another member of the international team. She had symptoms of a thyroid malignancy, and her skull tumour looked like it was a malignant metastasis. In hindsight, she seemed like a poor choice for neurosurgery. Without thyroid surgery, she would likely die of her throat disease long before her skull metastasis would affect her, but there was no one here who could operate on her thyroid.

During her surgery, the skull tumour turned out to be very bloody, and she used up the hospital's entire blood supply. A few of the nurses even gave blood in the operating room in a noble but futile effort to save her. The woman would die on a ventilator a few days later, never having regained consciousness. That one case also completely drained the hospital's oxygen supply. The next day's surgery was cancelled.

I now understood why we would do one case at a time.

On the third day, new oxygen tanks were delivered on the back of a pickup truck, red-tinged by the dust from the long drive from Monrovia. We were ready to go again.

I selected the young man with the brain tumour. The image of his tumour on the CT scan looked like a falx meningioma, a benign tumour that grows off the coverings of the brain and presses against the organ, causing dysfunction. If removed in its entirety, it could be cured. I did not yet know the patient's name when I met him in the male ward, where he was sitting in a wheelchair surrounded by his mother, wife and a small soccer team of his children.

The tumour was compressing the left side of his brain and causing paralysis of the right side of his body. He sat in his chair in front of the crowd of family members and was smiling asymmetrically at me, unable to stand or hold up his right arm. He seemed inappropriately happy for someone in hospital with a brain tumour. In his early thirties, he looked like a teenager with a beautiful, plump face; a young king sitting in his throne flanked by several rows of attendants. He smiled as if he owned the land we were standing on.

I stood immediately in front of him with an entourage of nurses, doctors and attendants fanning out behind me. My nurse translated after I spoke, and he would listen, pause as though it was a difficult question or he was giving the response serious consideration, and then respond.

I began, "How old are you?"

He replied at length with animated gestures of his left face and arm. More than a minute later, the nurse's translation came. "Thirty-two."

I hesitated but then asked, "Are you right- or left-handed?"

This time the response took several minutes. His voice was clear and deep. He spoke as if he was recounting a great historical tale, pausing for effect, then seeming to list off a series of points, each accentuated with finger counting. He eventually finished his narrative with a booming laugh suitable for a large man immensely pleased with himself. The translation came shortly thereafter. "Right."

Too impatient to risk another question, I asked the junior doctor to take his medical history after I examined him. He was five feet, eight inches and weighed 230 pounds. His right leg was completely paralyzed, his right arm was very weak, and the right side of his face did not move as well as the left when he smiled or spoke. However, his heart, lungs and vital signs were good. He would be a good candidate for surgery.

I asked the nurse for the surgical consent form. She had no idea what I was asking for, so I asked the junior doctor. He smiled and nodded, pretending to know what I was talking about, but did not move. Eventually it became clear that there was no such thing as a consent form. Patients accepted any and all treatments by virtue of the fact they were in hospital. I wrote my thoughts about his condition and my rationale for surgery in his chart and moved on.

The next morning, I met our brain tumour patient in the operating room. His name, Luogon Ouamouno, was handwritten on an identity band around his wrist. He smiled with the same peaceful confidence I'd observed the day before. The anaesthesiologist was very good, and Mr. Ouamouno was quickly asleep.

The surgery was enjoyable, with no surprises, except that the equipment we used would not have been out of place in the 1950s.

Nowadays we would typically use a high-speed drill to cut through the skull in seconds, but there were none available, so we cut through the bone with a hand drill and Gigli saw. The Gigli saw—a thin, flexible serrated wire held at each end by handles—is the most elegant instrument in neurosurgery, but it has not been in use in Canada for decades. The handles are pulled back and forth, allowing the wire to cut through bone.

Dr. Leonardo Gigli, a gynecologist from Italy, invented this saw in 1894 to cut the pubic bone during difficult labour. The saw was adopted by neurosurgeons a few years later and used extensively for almost a hundred years. Although praised around Europe, Gigli never received recognition from his Italian peers and died dejected at age forty-five. One researcher I met suggested he killed himself because of the deliberate snub, but the official version is much kinder: he died at home of pneumonia.

I quietly enjoyed the sweeping arm motion that maximized the saw's cutting. Most of neurosurgery is performed through small, precise finger movements. Under the microscope, I usually rest my hands on a support bar and just move the instruments between my thumb and index finger to isolate the normal physiological tremor of the arm from the instruments. The Gigli, however, invites exaggerated tai chi–like flowing movements from the shoulders. It is a careful dance that separates a piece of skull from the head and opens a window to the brain.

We hand-drilled four holes in Mr. Ouamouno's skull, one in each corner of a three-inch square. We then passed the Gigli wire under the skull from one hole to the next and connected the two handles. Alternately pulling each handle with long, fluid movements, I slowly sawed through the bone. Angling the wire down (not at right angles to the skull but at a shallow angle) produced a bevel on the edge of the bone. We repeated the cuts between each hole and soon had a square flap of bone with a bevelled edge that prevented it from being pushed into the brain.

The edges of the bone bled, and I asked for bone wax to seal it.

No one had heard of bone wax.

I gathered up the bone dust from the saw cuts and rubbed it over the bone edges to stop the bleeding. An old trick, but effective. The brain's covering, the dura, was stretched tight like a leather drum beneath the bone, and I began to cut through it to expose the under-lying brain. Running along the midline of the dura, over the top of his head, was a massive vein called the superior sagittal sinus that drains most of the blood from the brain at more than half a litre per minute. Mr. Ouamouno probably had just over seven litres of blood. Cutting this draining vein would cause torrential bleeding, and it was buried inside the dura near the top of our exposure. I cut the dura towards the sagittal sinus but stopped shorter than I normally would, just to be safe.

I asked how much blood was on hand in the blood fridge.

"None . . . and what's a blood fridge?" came the response. The stores had not been replenished since the first surgical disaster two days earlier.

I continued. No surgeon from Liberia had shown up, and I was very disappointed that no local doctor would learn from us and be equipped to carry on the work. At the time, however, there were only sixty doctors in the entire country. Perhaps it was too much to expect that one would be free to spend two weeks with us. In a short time, they would all be fighting a lethal virus.

I used my loops—black rim glasses with small magnifying lenses custom-built in—to see a magnified view of the surgical field. With the dura open, the brain was now visible. It was obviously distorted by a tan-grey rounded rock of tumour pushing into it.

I used a cutting cautery wire curved into a loop to burn and cut out scoops of the tumour. The wire was electrified at the touch of a button so it could burn through tissue, ideally cauterizing blood vessels as it went. The rock-hard tumour had knuckled into and distorted the soft brain. As the growth was shaved down, the brain relaxed and began to regain its natural shape. Eventually the entire tumour was removed, and the brain sagged back into the space the tumour had once occupied.

The tumour looked benign, not malignant. We did not have a pathologist to confirm this, but as I'd suspected, it looked like a meningioma, which is much firmer than the brain and pushes against it rather than infiltrating into it.

Mr. Ouamouno recovered quickly. The next day he was using his right arm to feed himself, and the following day he walked. He left the hospital to return to his village before the week was out. From my experience, his case was really straightforward. The only note of interest was the archaic surgical equipment.

The evening after Mr. Ouamouno's surgery, the medical team met in the air-conditioned room to discuss the next operation. We reviewed the two infants with massively enlarged heads characteristic of hydrocephalus. It was unheard of to see children like this in Canada—I had only seen images of such dramatically inflated heads in older textbooks. The two infant boys were similarly disfigured but had very different prognoses.

The first baby, Joshua, a nine-month-old, was otherwise healthy and happy. Hydrocephalus is a condition where the flow of cerebrospinal fluid (CSF) through the brain is blocked and the fluid builds up, ballooning the head. Descriptions of hydrocephalus date back to the father of medicine, Hippocrates (ca. 460–370 BCE); the word itself comes from the Greek words for "water" and "head." Dr. Walter

Dandy (whom we will meet in a future chapter) had begun to understand this condition almost a hundred years ago.

The CSF is a clear, water-like fluid that is produced within the ventricles (cavities) of the brain, and then flows through a series of these ventricles and eventually exits and flows around the organ. This allows the brain to float inside the skull rather than sit on the bottom of it. The CSF is finally absorbed into the superior sagittal sinus—but if there is a blockage anywhere along this route, the fluid builds up and the ventricles will massively dilate and crush the overlying brain against the inside of the skull. A baby's skull is made of separate bones that, to allow the brain to grow, do not fuse for several years. The gaps between these bones, fontanelles, feel like soft spots on the top of any baby's head. If hydrocephalus begins when the child is very young, before their skull has fused, the infant's head will balloon in size.

Before the 1950s, the condition or its attempted treatment was often lethal. In 1952, Dr. Eugene Spitz, a pediatric neurosurgeon at Children's Hospital in Philadelphia, placed a tube in the ventricle of a child with hydrocephalus and drained the CSF into her heart. The technique cured the hydrocephalus, but over-drainage of CSF, with the resultant rapid collapse of the brain and tearing of its blood vessels, caused the death of the child. A valve was needed in the tube to regulate the flow of CSF.

A few years later, one of Spitz's patients was Casey Holter, a child from Connecticut who was born with spina bifida and hydrocephalus. Casey's father, John, was a toolmaker. After talking to Spitz, he designed a one-way valve that could regulate the flow of CSF. Sadly Casey died eight days before his father made a working valve. Later John Holter would start a company that mass produced the Spitz-Holter shunt and ultimately saved thousands of lives.

Over the decades, treatments for hydrocephalus have evolved with our improved understanding of the condition and the human body. The original shunt procedure drained the excess fluid from the dilated ventricles in the brain through tubing into the jugular vein leading to the heart, but the body's immune reaction to the tubing produced antibodies that then clogged the kidney. The short-term miracle became a long-term death sentence by kidney disease. Now we place the lower end of the tubing in the peritoneum (the space between the outside of the bowels and the inside of the abdominal wall) to avoid long-term kidney damage.

Joshua had a CT scan that showed all his ventricles were enlarged and this was causing his brain to push outwards and enlarge his skull. He would benefit from a ventricular-peritoneal shunt, and I had brought one from Vancouver.

The second baby, also a boy, Saika, could not have been more different. Also nine months old, he could not lift his head off the crib where he lay. The brown skin of his scalp was stretched paper thin, and every vein was visible beneath its translucent surface. His mother was a young woman who only spoke Vai. She lived in a small village with no running water about three days' walk from the hospital, where she followed traditional customs and worship.

The name Saika means "the one who opened his mother"—a graphic description of a first-born. I was told he had been treated by the local healer, and when I asked for clarification, the nurse called him a witch doctor. When Saika's head began to grow, the healer wrapped it in a plaster of mud, manure and straw. The mixture baked in the sun, turned rock-hard and provided a helmet to limit further skull growth. Saika's head eventually broke open the plaster from the pressure of continued CSF accumulation, which must have been excruciatingly painful. I knew, as an outsider, that I held Western biases and should not judge, but when I heard this story and imagined the child's unnecessary suffering, I could not regard the traditional healer with equanimity.

Saika's CT head scan was so abnormal that it was difficult to pick out the normal structures. Most of Saika's brain was compressed by a grapefruit-sized cyst of fluid in the right side of his brain. All the ventricles were enlarged, and they were all pushed into the left side of the head. There was a small ribbon of abnormal brain surrounding everything, and the combination of the cyst fluid and enlarged ventricles had pushed the skull bones open, causing the massive head.

This was not someone who could be saved. That evening when we met to choose the next operation, the decision was clear: Joshua.

The following morning, Joshua had his surgery without incident. Everything went well and we were done by lunchtime. The follow-up CT showed the shunt was in an ideal location and had already begun to decompress his ventricles. Joshua was ready to go home in a few days. He would need a longer tube placed in his abdomen before his teenage growth spurt. That would be a problem if this operation did not become routine in Liberia during the next decade, so he was invited to come to Ghana if need be.

That afternoon, I played soccer with some high school boys on a field a few miles from the hospital. I'd brought a few T-shirts and gave them away to the winning team at the end of the game. The boys were quite skilled, despite the worn ball and uneven pitch, but when I had the ball, they were embarrassingly deferential. They did not tackle me unless the ball got a long way in front of me. Within ten minutes in the blistering heat, I was as soaked as a diver getting out of a pool. We shared the simple joy of running with a ball, and I briefly felt part of their world— not inserted there to help or instruct, but present there with all of them.

Our surgical team met again, later that evening, for supper and to discuss the next day's operation. To my surprise, the Nigerian neurosurgeon suggested we operate on Saika. I outlined why this would be futile.

Saika had a serious infection and we had no way of culturing the pathogen to choose the correct antibiotic. The infection probably came from the manure that had been wrapped around his head, the bacteria having entered through his thin scalp. We would not have strong enough antibiotics to handle an infection from bowel bacteria. Even if we did, we couldn't provide a long enough course of antibiotics.

A closer look at the images of his brain showed multiple smaller abscesses, and we had no way to drain them all. The infection would have already damaged his brain, and it was highly unlikely he would survive in his village. Some cases, like the woman with the malignant skull tumour, just could not be treated in this facility.

I was definitive in my assessment and categorical in my conclusion. We were not going to operate on Saika. This child was going to die and there was nothing any of us could do about it.

My colleague then began slowly to explain why I was mistaken. He was convinced we should operate and took great pains to support his case without saying my arguments were wrong. Unfortunately I had left no opening to consider an alternative, which clearly made him uncomfortable, since for his point to be considered, he would have to prove me wrong. Whereas I was accustomed to direct confrontation during management discussions, he was not.

"This child was born in a village where the local doctor is held in high esteem," he began. "His head grew unnaturally. The doctor tried to stop it, but he broke the doctor's treatment. He has now been taken away from them. The village will think he has been possessed and that there is some evil in his mother for her to have a child like this. She will be cast out of the village. We have to try to help them."

The doctor explained there were two reasons for proceeding. "In Africa, we are constantly faced with insurmountable difficulties when treating patients. It does not mean we should give up. We have to try and help, and be seen to try and help, even if we know the chances for survival are slim.

"Secondly, we have to try and help this boy so the village knows there was something medically wrong with him. We can fail, but they need to know we thought it was a medical problem. They are used to medicine failing. There is no cure for Ebola, for instance. If we stand back, they will think we believed there was something else wrong with him. They will cast the mother out. Even the poor child's mother will believe she has done something wrong to deserve this punishment."

Everyone in the room was nodding while he spoke. I was dumbstruck. I had never formulated a treatment around how society felt about a patient and his mother. They all looked at me. All I could say was, "Wow. I'd never thought about it like that." It did not take me long to come around to the idea that we would try to help this boy. The details of how we would do so, however, were unclear. It was medically unsound.

"What are you proposing we should do?"

"What would you recommend?" he replied.

"Wow."

That was all I could muster. I was flummoxed. I looked at Saika's CT scan again, which gave me a chance to think. Eventually I concocted what I considered to be a far-fetched but plausible plan. "We could try to drain the main fluid collection on the right side of the brain. He might get some temporary relief and we would be more certain of the diagnosis. If it is an abscess, we will know the prognosis is lethal."

"That is a grand plan," my colleague replied. "I will speak to

Mother." Tomorrow, Saika would get an operation. The Nigerian doctor had won his case.

We all assembled at 8 a.m. next to the operating room. I dressed in green scrubs and put on a pair of green rubber clogs. Operating room attire follows tradition more than scientifically proven hygienic practices. Studies have shown that people wearing street clothes shed less bacteria than those wearing surgical scrubs. One study showed that people who are naked shed less bacteria still. Even the surgical mask has not been shown to reduce surgical infections—its main function is to keep the patient's blood off the surgeon's face.

About the only thing that has been conclusively shown to reduce surgical infection is a sterile pair of gloves. In 1890 the aptly named Dr. Joseph Bloodgood showed that the surgeons at Johns Hopkins Hospital wearing sterile gloves had a lower infection rate than those who continued the tradition of operating bare-handed. It took thirty years for surgeons to catch on.

Saika arrived at 9 a.m.. He had been washed and changed by his mother and the nurse, and was carried into the anaesthetic room to get an IV. He was too weak to cry. He was laid on his back on a small table covered in green towels. His arms were outstretched and held by a nurse on one side and by the doctor who was looking for a vein on the other. His legs were frog-legged apart, which is normal for a newborn but not for an infant his age.

The room was very warm, ideal for Saika wrapped only in a small diaper, but I was sweating already. He could not move his massive head. His eyes were looking down, and I could just see the brown of his iris above his lower eyelid. This forced deviation of his eyes downwards, called sun-setting, is a common feature of severe hydrocephalus. His enlarged ventricles were squeezing the part of his brain responsible for lifting the eyes upwards.

There were no discernible veins in his arms or legs. The anaesthetist asked if he could use a scalp vein for the IV.

"Yes. But only on the left side," I said. "We will need the right side for our procedure."

While I was in bed the night before, I had thought about what we could do for Saika. Now I explained the plan to everyone in the room.

"We will hold him still, and I will put some local anaesthetic in his scalp. I will push a large needle through his scalp and between the splayed bones of his skull into where I think the abnormal fluid collection should be. I will then withdraw the plunger of the syringe and pull out whatever fluid is there. He is too sick to be put under a general anaesthetic, so we will just do it with some local." The brain does not feel pain when it is touched. Saika would not suffer as long as his scalp was numb from the local anaesthetic.

The most difficult part of the procedure was understanding where the fluid collection was located. I could see it on the CT scan but needed to translate those flat two-dimensional images into a three-dimensional understanding of his brain. The route to the fluid collection also needed to be between the skull bones, as I did not want to drill through his skull, which would require a large incision and entail dealing with bone bleeding (without bone wax) in a child with a very small blood volume.

I took a number of measurements off the CT and drew directly on Saika's head where I thought we should go through his scalp. I studied the images again to understand the depth and direction of the needle and how the fluid would then distort the brain after I began to remove it. Brain shift, with a needle deep inside the skull, could be disastrous.

When we were ready to begin, I asked to do a "WHO time out" but no one knew what that was. The World Health Organization has developed a safety checklist for patients having surgery. Prior to starting, the entire team reviews the patient's name (to ensure you have the correct patient), consent (to ensure you are doing the correct operation on the correct side), and a number of other factors that can be easily mistaken. I asked to see the consent form, but as before, there was none. That meant I would pass a needle freehand into Saika's head without the written consent of his mother. Although she understood we were trying to help, the nuances of how and why were clearly beyond her.

I gently washed Saika's scalp with warm soap and water for five minutes. The skin looked very fragile, and I did not scrub hard. I then washed his head with cotton swabs soaked in a dark brown iodine solution. We waited for the solution to dry.

The washing rubbed off my markings, but it was easy to remember where they were. I put a small amount of local anaesthetic under the skin with a tiny syringe. He did not cry. A nurse handed me a 60 cc syringe attached to a large-bore, 16-gauge needle that was three times thicker than his IV and two inches long. I bent over Saika, resting the back of my left hand on his head and holding the syringe in both hands.

"Okay, here we go," I announced. I oriented the large needle and syringe and then started to advance the sharp tip towards his skin.

That's precisely when the room lights went out, submerging us in complete darkness. It was early morning, but the operating room had no windows and was a few doors away from any source of natural light.

"What the hell?" the anaesthesiologist blurted.

I pulled back. I did not know where the sharp tip of my needle was, but I had not yet pierced Saika's head. All the monitors started to beep as they switched over to battery power. The noise was deafening, particularly in the dark. People were saying things to themselves and to the room at large, variations on "What's going on?" and "This is unacceptable."

About four or five minutes later, the lights came back on. Shortly after, someone in dirt-stained overalls peered around the doorway of the operating room and said, "Don't worry. We just switched over the generator."

The alarm on each monitor was eventually turned off, and gradually the operating room returned to normal. Saika continued to breathe, oblivious to the near disaster.

"Will you be turning off the generator again?" I asked the maintenance man.

"Yes. In twelve hours. Every day. Every twelve hours," he replied, then disappeared around the door.

I leaned over Saika again and advanced the needle towards his large head.

The steel needle pierced Saika's skin and penetrated deep into his brain. At the one-inch mark, I paused and continued to hold the syringe with my left hand resting on his head and pulled back the plunger with my right hand. The syringe filled with a thick green fluid. It was easy to get 50 cc. I twisted the syringe off the needle and put my left thumb over the exposed needle hub to stop anything being sucked back inside. I emptied the fluid into a kidney basin. It was not foul smelling, but it was definitely an abscess.

I reconnected the syringe and pulled out another 50 cc. Then another 50 cc, and another. I had estimated that the volume of the cyst before surgery was at least half a litre (500 cc). Saika's head began to collapse. The next pull of the syringe had resistance— something was blocking the flow of pus into the needle, probably the brain collapsing into the evacuated space. I withdrew the needle a bit and then repositioned it further backwards and deeper. The superficial part of the cyst had been evacuated; now I needed to get the deeper part. I pulled off another 50 cc and then stopped. I did not want a huge brain shift with the potential to tear some of his brain's vessels.

We would let the infant recover and then we would reimage his brain.

I put a small Band-Aid on his scalp where the needle had been. He was swaddled and bundled off to the recovery room and was back in his mother's arms a few hours later.

I went to see how Saika was doing with the medical team later that evening. His mother burst into tears when she saw us. She was crying with delight. Saika was much brighter and more active since surgery, she told me. He could cry with strength, and it sounded more like it used to before he couldn't lift his head up.

Everyone on our team was beaming and the mood was joyous. Everyone except me was truly happy.

I knew Saika would die in a few weeks.

I spoke to his mum through a nurse who translated. "We are all very proud of how strong Saika is and how well he did during surgery," I began. "He has an infection that made his head grow. I have removed some of the infection, but it is a strong infection and he is very young."

Usually when a translator is involved, both parties tend to address the translator. Now Saika's mum looked straight at me. Her eyes pierced mine and she spoke directly at me. "Can you do more?" came the translation from the nurse beside me.

"No," I replied, looking at the mother.

She bowed her head and turned away. She sat down in a chair beside the crib and looked at Saika and then up at me. "Thank you," came the translation. She did not cry or fuss. She picked him up and held him, rocking slightly back and forth with her son in her arms.

She understood.

Saika and his mum were welcomed back to their village a few days later. The nurses covered my small bandage with a very, very large dressing that wrapped around his head like a turban. It was clear to everyone that he had had a medical procedure—a brain operation.

Normally I get to see my patients after surgery in follow-up and learn how they did. Any problems are brought to my attention so a treatment plan and further care can be coordinated. Saika was a three days' walk away—I would not hear any further about him. I focused on the work ahead, but whenever it was quiet I found myself thinking about him.

The next week I did lumbar laminectomy operations on six elderly Liberians, one per day, removing the excess bone in their lower spine. The lumbar region is the lower back; laminectomy means to unroof the spinal canal. Each of them had severe spinal stenosis—a condition caused by constriction of the spinal canal by arthritic bone. The spinal canal protects the spinal nerves to the lower limbs, but if the canal is choked with arthritic bone, there is no room for the nerves and they are crushed into malfunction. Patients can no longer walk more than a block at a time. They must stoop forwards to try and relieve the pressure. The cure is simple: remove the bone covering the canal and change a constricted circle into an open trough.

Each operation was technically easy but physically demanding. Crunching through the arthritic bone with a dull rongeur, the pliers-like surgical instrument for gouging out bone, was fatiguing on my hands. The anaesthesiologist was amazed that the procedure could be done without a blood transfusion. At his institute, patients routinely got several units of blood. In Vancouver this was unheard of. A clean dissection of the muscle off the bone before removing the bone reduced the blood loss. Unfortunately no Liberian surgeon would learn this during my visit.

As the time to depart Tappita approached following our two-week stay, more news of Ebola began to emerge. The airlines into Monrovia started to cancel flights. For the first time, I started to get very nervous. No longer distracted by the business of planning and doing surgery, I was free to worry about the actual risk of infection.

On our drive back to Monrovia, we stopped at a bridge between Liberia and Guinea near the village of Meliandou, where the first Ebola victim, a two-year-old boy called "patient zero" by the scientists, had died. The deadly virus spread from this Guinean toddler to his family and then to the Liberian woman who walked across the border and died in Foya. The bridge was patrolled by soldiers wearing paper masks and no gloves. I gave them two boxes of thick blue vinyl gloves and a small supply of N95 masks, and they were immensely grateful. The N95 mask can protect against airborne pathogens like COVID-19 or influenza; Ebola is not spread through the air but by direct touching contact with the virus, which made the gloves especially valuable. The local ritual of kissing and washing the dead bodies of relatives inadvertently helped spread the disease. Unfortunately, when the WHO criticized these local customs, it only spread mistrust among some of the people of Liberia.

The Liberian captain was very pleased to escort me across the yellow metal bridge over the St. John River into Guinea, where we met his counterpart and the Guinean soldiers guarding the entrance into their country. I gave them a box of gloves and spoke to them briefly, in French, explaining why we were there. They saluted us, then we crossed back and were off to Monrovia.

When I arrived, I ate dinner in the hotel and waited in my locked room for the plane to come the next day from London. Flights in and out of Monrovia were being cancelled on an ad hoc basis. The news was sparse and unreliable. Eventually Air France, Delta and British Airways would stop flying into Monrovia altogether.

My flight from London did arrive—I had never been so happy to see an airplane. The British Airways jet was parked in the middle of the tarmac, dwarfing the small propeller planes beside it. When I boarded it was obvious that the cabin crew were equally jubilant to be leaving. Apparently they had had an unwelcomed layover in Monrovia. We departed without incident. Normally I would be nervous during take-off, but this time, when the twin engines roared and pushed me back into my seat, I was too tired to care.

More than five hundred Liberian doctors, nurses and midwives would die in this Ebola outbreak, including the head surgeon of the Redemption Hospital in Monrovia. No one from our team became infected, probably because of our relatively short time there and the nature of our work. It is the front-line workers who risk exposure to Ebola or COVID-19, not the neurosurgeons operating on one person at a time inside a sterile room.

I was continuing my life, but Saika would soon be slipping away from his. His brief time in this world was painful, but he would surely die in his mother's arms, surrounded by members of his village who no longer believed he was possessed by evil spirits. I could not put into words why I felt I was a better doctor for having met him. I only knew it was so.

Saika and his mother (whose name I never learned) stayed in my thoughts after I returned to Canada and the safety of my predictable life. I kept returning to them. I gradually allowed myself to admit that one of the reasons I had been reluctant to operate on Saika was that I knew I would lose. He was going to die and I would fail to save him— and I was afraid of that failure. After almost twenty years as a neurosurgeon at that point, no patient of mine had ever died after an elective operation. I had never confided this to anyone, but I did not want that winning streak to end. It was a selfish obsession. At that time, I valued my work more as a technician than as a healer. My goal was to remove the tumour without complication rather than improve the patient's life. Saika taught me to see purpose in helping the patient but losing to the disease. He also taught me that healing the patient occurs within the context of their society, not within the isolation of their illness.

From then on I relearned this lesson repeatedly in my career—no more so than when one of my patients told me, "You fixed my Parkinson's but ruined my life!" I had eliminated his Parkinsonian disability with a deep brain stimulation (DBS) operation, but his wife, who had only remained with him because of a sense of duty to nurse him, divorced him. He was able to be physically independent but now desperately hated the prospect.

Saika also taught me that even after years of study, training and practice, I could be completely wrong. My African colleagues knew what to do: try to save a life. Operating on Saika provided evidence to his village that his death was not due to evil spirits, thereby liberating his mother from a life of exclusion, castigation and shame. Social progress was made. A life *was* saved. Saika's mother's life. My co-workers had made the right call.

On the flight back to Europe, still mentally immersed in the drama, I reclined my seat as we reached cruising altitude. What had just happened? My nerves were jangled. I had a glass of sparkling wine, my first drink in two weeks, hoping it might relax me. The carbon dioxide bubbles in the champagne allowed the alcohol to enter my bloodstream directly from the stomach, rather than from lower in the gut. It was the perfect aperitif, also the fastest. I found myself thinking back over my career.

How the heck had I ended up in Liberia? The lines from Robert Frost's famous poem entered my head:

Two roads diverged in a wood, and I—
I took the one less traveled by,
And that has made all the difference.

That struck me as an apt metaphor for my journey. First I had opted to be a surgeon, the less-travelled road among physicians. Then at a later fork in the road, I'd chosen neurosurgery. I can remember first wanting to become a brain surgeon when I was in grade six. Though I was completely naive about what it really meant, the idea of neurosurgery was somehow appealing, and I loved drawing pictures of the brain. The actual moments when I had to choose one road or the other came much later.

Now safely in a plane among the clouds, I recalled the very case that had crystallized my decision to be a surgeon. I was an intern in the emergency department of St. Michael's Hospital in Toronto when I suddenly knew with absolute certainty the path I would follow. I had long intended to write about that pivotal moment someday. My mind was still racing from Liberia; I couldn't sleep. The flight back to London would give me almost seven hours.

I started writing about Jeff.

2.

JEFF, THE MAN WHO DIED
TWICE AND LIVED

I t is not uncommon to remember a patient because of an unexpected complication. This is how the practice of medicine slowly
improves. The poor results of a mistaken diagnosis or a misguided
treatment help to inform you how to change your future treatments.
These patients change how we practise medicine, but they do not alter
our world view.

Occasionally, however, you will meet a patient who changes you as
a person. Someone who changes your core beliefs, your motivation or
your understanding of the world. In the fall of 1986, I encountered a
young man who crystallized my decision to study surgery.

I was an intern at St. Michael's Hospital in Toronto, having just
finished medical school at the University of Toronto and begun a one-
year clinical rotation to complete my medical qualifications. In those
days, you needed an internship before you could get a licence to practise medicine. Qualified doctors then either started a family practice
or went on to further training in a medical specialty as a resident.
Many family practitioners objected to the concept that you were either
a specialist or a family doctor—they felt they were also specialists.

A residency program for specialization in family practice was started, and internships disappeared.

After medical school, students must now enter a residency. Unfortunately, they must choose which residency they will apply for during their third year. Some do not yet know what interests them, and some get stuck in the wrong specialty.

Back in the 1980s, a medical student who had chosen to specialize had to decide between medicine or surgery. Medicine was the world of cardiologists, endocrinologists and neurologists. Surgery was the world of cardiac surgeons, general surgeons and neurosurgeons. I knew I was interested in the brain and its function (who isn't?), but the day-to-day life of a surgeon was a complete mystery to me. As a naive ten-year-old, I had found neurosurgery appealing, but now, a medical intern at age twenty-five, I was learning the realities of that lifestyle. I was on call for the first time, working all night and then continuing through the next day. I began to have doubts and to question whether it was actually the right path for me.

That doubt was allayed one night in the emergency room of St. Michael's Hospital.

St. Mike's, as it is known, is a downtown Toronto teaching hospital on Queen Street just east of Yonge. It was established by the Catholic Sisters of St. Joseph in 1892 with the goal of looking after the sick and poor of the inner city. Its location ensured a steady clientele coming in from living rough on the streets.

In my experience, these patients often had advanced disease when they arrived. They received their care for free and, in turn, were excellent patients for teaching medicine. Their illnesses were so obvious, even an intern could recognize them. Many of the homeless patients had mental illness and addiction problems, with alcohol featuring prominently. Alcohol in excess will damage the liver, and a damaged liver causes abdominal pain, nausea and anorexia in mild cases. Moderate damage causes jaundice (yellow skin), ascites (excess fluid in the belly) and swollen legs. The patients at St. Mike's often had severe damage, with liver cirrhosis and all of its protean accompanying signs. I had memorized at least a dozen of these signs, including a few rare ones.

Alcohol can cause hypogonadism in men (shrunken testicles) with resultant gynecomastia ("man boobs") and feminization of hair. With a reduction of the male hormone, testosterone, there was no male-pattern baldness. In fact, these men often had luxuriously beautiful, though unkempt, hair. Boris Yeltsin, the Russian president before Putin, was as famous for his beautiful hair as for his reported drunkenness.

The patients at St. Mike's were also often involved in violent altercations—mostly with each other, but occasionally with the police. I learned how to suture by closing the faces and hands of these inner-city warriors. When my fiancée, Karla, and I would go out for dinner on the weekend, we would often walk past one of these folks and I would recognize my handiwork.

"See the scar on that man's face above his right eye?" I would quietly whisper to her as we walked along Queen Street. "I did that one last week." Occasionally I would get a "Hey, Doc" and a knowing nod as we passed by.

St. Mike's was a level-one trauma centre, meaning it took the most severely injured. The other level-one trauma centre was Sunnybrook Hospital. Located close to Toronto's main expressway, Highway 401, it therefore received the lion's share of motor vehicle accidents. We got the urban trauma. Knife fights, gunshots and good, old-fashioned beatings.

I had chosen St. Mike's for my internship because the chair of neurosurgery at the University of Toronto worked there. He had called me into his office when I was a medical student and said, "You will apply to our program. And nowhere else." He knew I was interested in neurosurgery, and by that time I had accepted a Rhodes scholarship to do a doctoral degree in neurophysiology at Oxford after my internship. I replied with complete sincerity, "Why would I go elsewhere?" It truly had never occurred to me that there might be other places to study medicine or neurosurgery. At that time, Toronto was the centre of the universe for me.

After a few years in Oxford, however, it became clear that there were other places to live, and we never did return to Toronto. Karla thought that Vancouver was the most beautiful city and that was it. We moved to Vancouver, where I did my neurosurgical residency, and before I had finished, I was offered a job at the University of British Columbia.

My internship was designed to provide a generalized exposure to a variety of specialties. I spent two months each in the emergency, obstetrics, pediatrics, internal medicine, psychiatry and surgery departments.

The most interesting patients turned out to be on the psychiatry ward and in their outpatient clinics. I met a manic middle-aged woman who brought the staff a layered cake each week she visited the clinic. The degree of her mania correlated directly with the number of layers in her cake, and her psychiatrist titrated her dose of lithium to keep the layers below four. Lithium is a naturally occurring salt that can be found dissolved in some spring water. San Pellegrino, for example, has some lithium, while Perrier does not. The chemical has been concentrated and used as a mood stabilizer for over a hundred years without us knowing exactly how it works.

Mania is the opposite of depression, and some researchers believe it is the brain's defence against depression. The two polar opposite conditions can co-exist in the same patient in a condition called bipolar disorder (what used to be called manic depression). The classic features of mania are seen in over-the-top behaviour: a larger-than-life personality, completely self-assured, loud, colourful, but out of touch with reality. If happy is to the right of neutral on a theoretical mood scale, euphoria would be even further right, and mania would be beyond that, though it's difficult to define where "normal" jubilation ends and "abnormal" mania begins. When your behaviour causes you to do things that consistently hurt you, it is probably abnormal.

Our manic patient in the psychiatry clinic was always a pleasure, full of life and ready to entertain. Most people enjoy meeting someone who is manic, but the condition can detach the patient from reality and become dangerous. One day she arrived dressed completely in red. Red hat and earrings, red socks and shoes, red dress, and perhaps the brightest red lipstick I had ever seen. It was impossible not to smile when you met her. Clearly abnormal, but exuding happiness and joy. A good defence against depression.

During my time on the psychiatry ward, I met profoundly depressed patients for the first time. Their symptoms were distinct from all other medical conditions I had seen—many of these patients had lost all hope and had given up trying to be well. Most patients with a severe illness continue to fight the disease and try to recover or adapt; even patients who become severely disabled from cancer or trauma continue to have the human will to survive. The profoundly depressed, however, lose that part of their humanity. They are lost and indifferent; they have learned helplessness.

My time with the psychiatrists themselves, however, felt like show and tell. The psychiatrist said the patient had one diagnosis, but I could not distinguish that patient's symptoms from the next one who had a completely different diagnosis. Either the field was way over my head, or the psychiatrists' diagnostic confidence was misplaced. Not my cup of tea.

The pediatric ward taught me that children were not just little adults, they had different physiology and diseases. Unfortunately, the care of these patients was dominated by the interactions with their parents. Ten minutes examining a child and half an hour explaining the results to the mother. Not my cup of tea.

The obstetrical ward was like war. The trench warfare of the First World War has been described as "months of boredom punctuated by moments of extreme terror"—that was also an apt description of my duties on the obstetrical ward. I remember being very excited when my first patient went into labour, only to slowly lose interest over the next two days of sleepless nights. The nurse eventually delivered the child and left me sleeping. When I was awake, it seemed the infants were born despite my ignorance of how to deliver them—I just caught them before they hit the floor. Not my cup of tea.

My internal medicine rotation was with an endocrinologist for one month and then a nephrologist for another. They were both brilliant, far smarter than any neurosurgeon I had met. They understood every aspect of the diseases they treated. They examined, they tested and they pre-scribed. They re-evaluated, they ruminated and they prescribed. They mused, they cogitated and they prescribed. But the intellectual chal-lenge was never balanced with any physical action. Not my cup of tea.

My surgery rotation began with one month of general surgery. It was underwhelming. My chief resident talked me through an appen-dectomy during my first week, and instead of being elated that I had done the entire operation myself, I was disappointed that an operation could be completed by someone who had never seen it done with just a few words of guidance. I imagined I would become comfortably numb by my hundredth case.

During the second week, I was scheduled to assist at the incision and drainage of a peri-anal abscess. To this day, it is the only operation I have seen that made me nauseous. The obese patient was asleep on his back under a general anaesthetic with his legs spread-eagled in stirrups—as if he might give birth. The abscess, bulging and red, distorted his anus into a crescent moon. The senior resident sat on a stool between the patient's legs, at eye level with the abscess, charged with the responsibility of cutting the skin over it to allow the pus to escape. He paused and I felt the first throes of nausea. He began to speak instead of just slashing the skin. Serious nausea welled up. He then pontificated on the correct instrument and technique to perform this ridiculously simple procedure. My stomach tightened.

"Some might think that this procedure requires . . ." he said. I began retching and had to leave. I can't remember if I ran or walked out, but there was vomit in my mouth. I ripped off my mask and spat into the scrub sink outside the OR, feeling sweaty, dizzy and faint. Definitely not my cup of tea.

My time on the neurosurgery service was also not particularly inspiring. I was at the bottom of the pecking order and did most of the scut work—all the routine and boring work that no one else wanted to do. Shit flows downhill. I certainly did not do any operations; instead, I spent most of my time on the ward dealing with the medical issues of chronic patients so that the residents would not be disturbed in the OR. Going through the motions but not enjoying a single moment of my time.

I began to flounder in an ocean of indecision regarding my future. None of the specialties had interested me so far. Even neurosurgery had been disappointing. There was no spark, no passion, no drive.

I was lost.

My time on the emergency service turned out to be very interesting. There were so many different conditions that every case was my first. The interns were given a lot of autonomy in those days. The charge nurse would hand you a clipboard and tell you to go see a particular patient; you would meet them, listen to their history and examine them, order whatever tests you wanted and then have to make a diagnosis. Then you would call in the emergency room physician and present the case to them. It was a cerebral exercise and I felt that it really mattered. Finally I was actually helping someone.

Most of the cases were straightforward: an exacerbation of asthma or the latest episode of angina. Some were sad: a fifteen-year-old prostitute with florid gonorrhea, or the ubiquitous pneumonia of someone living on the streets. Some were exciting: a cardiac arrest or a stabbing. Some were frightening: a psychotic event in a shackled prisoner or perhaps a child who could not breathe. Each case came during an eight- or twelve-hour shift. It was interesting work, but it was just work. None of these patients changed my perspective on life or confirmed my choice of specialty. Until I met Jeff Sageman.

When he first arrived in the emergency department, he was identified as "Unknown Male C"—the third unknown male that day. He was a nineteen-year-old construction worker who had fallen twenty feet off a scaffolding while installing windows in the new L'Hôtel. The paramedics had found him on his back, unconscious but breathing, and had transported him to St. Mike's on a spine board with a neck collar.

I saw him get wheeled into the trauma bay surrounded by a crowd of medical people scuttling sideways to keep up with the stretcher. He was lifted onto the gurney with great care not to move his back in case he had a spinal injury. The bones in your back form a protective casing around the spinal cord, and if the spine is broken, the bones may move unduly and cut or damage the spinal cord, permanently paralyzing the patient. The bones of a broken spine can be fixed, but damage to the spinal cord cannot.

My pager went off and the shrill beeps continued until I pressed it quiet. I was part of the trauma team that day and was being summoned into the trauma bay. The physician in charge was Grant Drysdale, an emergency doctor in his early fifties, short, lean, with grey frizzled hair puffing out from the sides of his head and a bald spot on top. He wore a white lab coat, undone and with pockets filled with instruments, over his white shirt and an unfashionably wide tie. Ties would not become taboo in medical environments for another decade, after several studies showed they had more bacteria than toilet seats. Dr. Drysdale had very large dark rim glasses with obvious bifocal lenses and looked like an older detective Lieutenant Columbo but balding. He was standing at the bottom of the gurney and was getting the story from a paramedic.

"Unknown male had a witnessed fall. Fell backwards about twenty feet. Off a scaffold. Landed on the ground. No medical history. Vitals stable. BP 130 on 80. Heart rate 120. Respiratory rate 24. Afebrile. Glasgow score was 3 at the scene but 14 in the ambulance," the paramedic rattled off. The Glasgow Coma Scale, developed by two Scottish neurosurgeons in the 1970s, is a numeric representation of the level of consciousness. It was a welcomed replacement for the colourful but vague terms "stuporous," "drowsy," and "somnolent." The scale ranges from 3, deeply comatose, to 15, fully alert. Although initially criticized for starting at 3 instead of 0, it has become the worldwide standard. Our patient was a 14/15, which means he was alert but confused.

Unknown Male C was being attacked on all sides. The orderly ran an open pair of large, orange-handled scissors up one pant leg; his jeans tore open against the blades without any scissoring until the waistband. A moment later, his shirt was flayed open and he lay naked on the gurney. He fought with everyone.

He was in obvious pain and moaning loudly with each breath through clenched teeth. His eyes were closed—not passively closed from unconsciousness, but actively squeezed shut from the pain. I could see he was moving all four limbs, which was a good sign: it meant he did not have an obvious spinal cord injury. I knew his spine could still be broken, though. In fact, 5 percent of spinal cord injuries occur after arrival to the hospital, when the broken spine is not recognized and subsequent movements of the patient allow the broken bone to cut into the soft spinal cord.

Unknown Male C lay on a thin, hard wooden spine board on top of the gurney and had a hard-plastic white cervical collar around his neck. Both the board and collar were to keep his spine immobilized.

There is a particular choreography to the sequence of events amid the chaos of treating a trauma victim. There may be minor changes in the order, but the lead physician conducts each step, cueing the nurses, orderlies and interns. Dr. Drysdale was in charge and he was comfortable in the position. His calm forcefulness radiated into the other team members. It is a pleasure to work under the guidance of someone whom you trust will catch you if you fall. I stood behind Dr. Drysdale, waiting to be told what to do.

The nurses, one on each side of the patient, pushed IVs into his arms. "Large-bore IV is in," both said almost simultaneously.

"What gauge?" asked Drysdale.

"Sixteen," responded the first nurse.

"Same," responded the second. They moved to their next tasks: sticking electrocardiogram leads on his chest and putting a small white pulse oximeter on his finger. The monitor began to beep with each heartbeat at a pitch that was proportional to the amount of oxygen in his blood. The beep had a reassuringly high pitch. A blood pressure cuff was wrapped around his upper right arm and immediately began to inflate and squeeze his arm to take the first reading.

A third nurse was "charting," writing everything down on a flow sheet. His blood pressure was 105/55; lower than it should be but not alarming. His heart rate was 130 and his respiratory rate was 26; both higher than normal but not surprising for a patient in pain.

Within the next half-hour, Unknown Male C would die—twice.

Drysdale assessed the victim's airway, breathing and circulation. The A, B, Cs of resuscitation. Everything was okay. He had an open airway leading to his lungs, his lungs sounded like they were filling with air, and his blood was circulating with a reasonable pressure. To protect the victim's spine, Drysdale was careful not to move him or his collar.

The next step in the sequence was D for disability. Drysdale could see the victim was moving all his limbs. He spoke to him, "Can you tell me your name?"

Drysdale moved right beside the victim's face and spoke again, a bit louder, "Can you tell me your name?"

Unknown Male C spoke through his clenched teeth, "Jeff . . ."

"Jeff, where does it hurt?"

"My back, my back, my fuckin' back." The words were muffled, but it was clear to everyone where and how much pain he had.

"I'm going to examine you to make sure you don't have any broken bones," Drysdale continued. He moved quickly through Jeff's scalp, face and jaw and then bypassed his collared neck to his chest and abdomen, before methodically squeezing up and down each arm and leg.

"We need to roll him," he announced, and all the players took their positions. Everyone stood on Jeff's right side except Drysdale. One nurse held the head, another reached across his chest to hold his left arm, the orderly reached across his legs to hold his left thigh, and I stood motionless not knowing what to do.

Drysdale looked at me and said, "Grab his legs." I moved beside the orderly and held Jeff's ankles. Drysdale counted, "On three. Ready, one . . . two . . . three." In a manoeuvre called the log roll, everyone rolled Jeff sideways towards them so Dr. Drysdale could see his back while keeping the spine immobile and in a straight line.

Drysdale leaned over and palpated firmly and methodically all the way down Jeff's back from below the collar to his tailbone. He stood up and said, "Jeff, I have to put a gloved finger in your rectum." That examination was quick. "Good rectal tone," he said to the charting nurse. Loss of rectal tone (the tension keeping the anus closed) is a sign of spinal cord injury. Drysdale took off his soiled left glove and stood upright.

"Wait a second. What's that?" He was still looking at Jeff's back.

"There's a one-inch cut between the ribs on the left," he dictated for the nurse scribe. He probed it with his still-gloved right hand. "There's something stuck in it."

"Hold still and give me another glove," he commanded. We were holding Jeff at an angle so the left side of his back was lifted off the spine board but his spine remained straight. It was easy for me because I was holding his ankles, but the nurse holding his upper body was struggling a bit.

Drysdale reached back into the thin slit of a wound and found a piece of glass. He started pulling it out and Jeff moaned louder. I could not see what was happening; none of us could because we were on the other side holding Jeff up. Drysdale's head was bent low, focused on the incision. I thought I heard him say "holy shit" but it was not clear. Whatever he was saying, he kept repeating it, over and over. Then he stood up straight and held up a bloodied shard of glass. It was at least six inches long.

"Oh, happy dagger!" Drysdale held up the stiletto to show us all. It was as long as a steak knife and only slightly wider.

"Roll him back," he said quietly. ". . . and call thoracics!" he yelled out to the charting nurse. The volume of his voice underlined the urgency of his request for the thoracic surgery team, who dealt with serious chest injuries.

We slowly rolled Jeff back down. The moment he lay flat on his back, he went limp. He stopped moaning and his arms fell to his sides. Still holding onto his ankles, I noticed his feet, which had been pointing straight up, now flopped open to the sides.

"Holy shit." This time Dr. Drysdale's words were crystal clear. "What's his pressure?"

The nurse inflated the blood pressure cuff and, after what seemed like an eternity, said, "I've got nothing."

Drysdale demanded two litres of saline "statum!" He was both a Shakespearean and a Latin scholar—*statum* meant immediately but was usually shortened to "stat" by the medical plebeians. He also called for "Four units of O-neg." O-negative blood is the universal blood donor type that can be given to anyone.

Give A+ blood to someone who is O-, and they can die. The immune system of the recipient O- patient has never seen the A antigen, and therefore attacks it because it is foreign. Give O- blood to someone who is A+, however, and everything is fine. The O- means there are no A or B antigens in the blood (the O stands for zero); therefore, the recipient's immune system sees nothing foreign to attack.

Drysdale did not know Jeff's blood type, but he knew he could give him O- blood, which was always kept in the blood fridge for emergencies. It arrived in the hands of a breathless orderly and was soon hanging on an IV pole and pouring into Jeff's left arm.

Drysdale was visibly shaken. Unknown Male C was in trouble, and he had about five minutes to figure out the problem before his patient would die. He defaulted to the trauma protocol, hoping the solution would reveal itself, beginning again with the primary survey of the A, B, C, Ds (airway, breathing, circulation, disability) followed by a thorough secondary examination of each body system.

Jeff was deeply unconscious, motionless and unresponsive. Drysdale, standing on the patient's left side, grabbed his shoulder, squeezed it and yelled at him, "Jeff, open your eyes!" There was no response. He grabbed Jeff's left nipple, squeezed and turned it, and yelled again, "Does that hurt?" Nothing. The nurse clenched her jaw reflexively. Without any blood pressure to perfuse Jeff's brain, it had stopped working. Drysdale looked at her. "We'll tube him. Give me an 'eight.'"

Drysdale was going to intubate the patient, because an unconscious person cannot keep their airway open. They do not "swallow their tongue," but the tongue can relax back in the throat and cut off the airway to the lungs. Drysdale moved around to the head of the bed, opened Jeff's mouth with a metal-bladed laryngoscope and slid a number 8 sized endotracheal tube down his throat. Jeff gave no resistance, and the tube was connected to a ventilator to breathe for him.

Four minutes left.

Drysdale listened to the patient's chest with his stethoscope. With each pump of the ventilator, he could hear the air filling both lungs. There was no problem with airway or breathing. Circulation, however, was catastrophically impaired. "What's his pressure?"

"Nothing," the nurse responded. She had been wanting to tell Drysdale that crucial fact but waited until she was asked. The team was following protocol closely. I stepped back away from the foot of the bed to stay out of the way but ready to help when told what to do. This was no longer a learning moment where a mentor would stop to teach you some important point. A life was slipping away and only Drysdale could save him. We were his extra pairs of hands, not his partners.

Three minutes.

"Why's he got no pressure?" Drysdale verbalized his thoughts. No one answered; it was obvious he was asking only himself. He glanced up at the ECG (electrocardiogram) tracing that looked like a flat line to him from where he was standing.

"Start compressions," he commanded, and the team immediately moved to begin CPR—cardiopulmonary resuscitation. The bed was lowered and the nurse on Jeff's right side stood up on a footstool and leaned down on the patient's chest with both her arms straight, hands on top of one another with her fingers clasped. She leaned the heel of her hands hard into the middle of Jeff's chest and counted, "One and two and three and four, and five and six and seven and eight. . ." Each compression pushed Jeff's chest down against his spine and squeezed his heart, mimicking a heartbeat. The compressions forced whatever blood was in his heart to move out into the aorta and around his body, thanks to its one-way valve system.

"Good compressions," Drysdale announced unemotionally. This was a confirmation of the depth of chest compressions, not a compliment. Too-shallow compressions did not move enough blood; too-deep broke the ribs. After fifteen compressions, the respiratory therapist squeezed the ventilation bag and pushed two large breaths into the patient's lungs. The endotracheal tube had been disconnected from the ventilator and attached to a bag of oxygen so the breaths could be coordinated with the chest compressions. After thirty compressions, another two breaths.

"Hold compressions." Drysdale reached for the patient's neck and the team remained motionless. He tried to find Jeff's carotid pulse to see if his heart was working, and moved his fingers around above the hard neck collar in several places. Drysdale looked up at the ECG rhythm and saw a flat line. In reality, there was a faint trace of a heart rhythm, but Drysdale could not see it because the monitor was above his head and his bifocals showed him only details that were below his nose.

Two minutes.

"Restart compressions." He could not find a pulse.

The nurse resumed her compressions and the respiratory therapist waited for her moment to squeeze the bag.

"Asystole." Drysdale called out the heart rhythm he saw on the monitor. A flat line meant no heartbeat—asystole. Once the rhythm was defined, the treatment was predetermined by the trauma protocol. Each abnormal heart rhythm, or arrhythmia, had a prescribed treatment.

"Give me a shot of 'epi' and be prepared to shock him." Drysdale called for the defibrillator and the nurse injected one milligram of epinephrine into the IV. Epinephrine is the injectable form of adrenalin, the powerful hormone behind the "flight or fight" response that kicks the heart with a boost of energy. Drysdale knew asystole would not respond to a defibrillator shock, but he must have wanted to be ready in case the rhythm changed to something that was shockable.

The nurse pushed down on Jeff's chest and the respiratory therapist blew air into his lungs. Drysdale held Jeff's wrists to measure the degree of pulsation in his radial artery. "Deeper compressions," Drysdale commanded. The nurse put the full weight of her shoulders into the compressions, but the doctor could not feel much pulsation.

"Deeper!" Drysdale was not pleased, but the nurse was maxing out on her effort.

"Chris! Take over compression." He flashed a glance at me. I moved beside the nurse ready to crush Jeff's chest. My own adrenalin had charged my muscles and potentially inflated my impression of how well I could do.

I began compressions, "One and two and three and four . . ." counting up to fifteen and then a pause for the two breaths. I was standing on the footstool and staring straight ahead at the ECG monitor only a few feet in front of me.

After a few cycles Drysdale said, "Hold compressions!" and we froze in position. I stared at the monitor and saw a faint tracing of a pulse. It had the characteristic shape of an ECG tracing, but the amplitude was reduced almost to a flat line.

"Asystole," Drysdale called out. "Resume compressions."

"No!" I shouted. "He has a rhythm."

"What?" Drysdale was as surprised that I would contradict him as he was that I thought there was a rhythm. The room was silent. The protocol does not allow for discussion or dissent. Everyone was staring at me, but I just looked at Drysdale and spoke directly to him.

"There's a rhythm, I can see it," I assured him.

He moved right up to the monitor and lifted his glasses and tilted his head way back.

"Agree," he announced. He was calmer than I was and emotionless in his tone. There was no "Congratulations!" or "How dare you?" It was just the right answer and now the protocol changed.

"EMD," Drysdale called out. "Another shot of epi.'"

Electromechanical dissociation, or EMD, occurs when there is some electrical activity in the heart but no coordinated pulsation to push any blood. The chance of survival is 20 percent.

One minute.

"Resume compressions," Drysdale ordered, and I leaned down hard on Jeff's chest. We began another cycle when the doctor yelled "Stop!" We froze and looked at him. This was outside the protocol. No one knew what to do next.

In a flash of intuition, Drysdale had suddenly understood exactly what was happening to Jeff. He pulled open the stiff cervical collar around the patient's neck.

Jeff's neck veins were engorged with blood, standing out like ropes under his skin. Drysdale was directly opposite me. He turned to look at me over the top of his glasses and said, "Cardiac tamponade!"

The diagnosis explained everything and, more importantly, had a treatment. The heart is surrounded by an empty sac called the pericardium, which allows the heart to beat without rubbing into anything else. If the sac fills with blood, however, the heart is squeezed smaller. It can still beat but it cannot fill with much blood between each beat. The output of the heart, its pulse, gets weaker and weaker until the heart cannot fill at all. The electrical activity continues but its ECG signal is muffled by all the surrounding blood into a dampened wiggle.

The glass dagger had cut into Jeff's heart but had plugged its own hole. When the dagger was removed, the ruptured heart began squirting blood into the pericardial sac, choking the muscle closed. The cure was to relieve the pressure around the heart by draining the fluid in the pericardial sac.

"Cardiocentesis needle," Drysdale ordered, and the nurse flew to the shelves at the back of the trauma bay and returned with a small rectangular box wrapped in sterile green cloth.

Drysdale looked at me and said, "Sterile gloves. Prep the belly." He opened the tray and put it between Jeff's legs as I gloved and rubbed Jeff's lower chest and abdomen with brown iodine, which pooled in his belly button. I wondered why he was asking me to be involved at this crucial stage. Perhaps it was a small reward for seeing the rhythm.

Drysdale connected the cardiocentesis syringe to an unimaginably long needle—it was at least a foot long. He attached one of the ECG wires to the needle with an alligator clip and then turned to me. "Stand here. Enter here. Aim for his right shoulder." Drysdale was pointing to a spot just below Jeff's lowest left rib.

I was stunned that he wanted me to do this but immediately walked around to Jeff's left side and took hold of the mother of all needles, then pushed its tip into Jeff's skin below his rib exactly where Drysdale had pointed. The skin puckered inwards, then gave way as the needle plunged through. I was aiming for Jeff's shoulder, and his heart was somewhere along the way.

"When you feel the heart, stop and suck back." Drysdale's instructions were simple, but I had no idea what the heart would feel like at the end of a long needle.

"If the ECG fires, you're in too deep," he added. That made sense because the needle would cause the heart to fire and we would see that electricity with an ECG wire connected to the needle.

Unexpectedly, I did feel the needle push on the pericardial sac and then pop through. "I think I got it," I said and started to pull back on the plunger. Everyone in the room was silent and staring at the syringe. I pulled harder on the plunger. It stuck momentarily and then gave way and glided back. Dark red blood flowed easily into the barrel. After 30 cc, the plunger stopped. It was sucking against something and no more blood came.

Jeff sat bolt upright.

The needle was still six inches into his chest. I let go of the blood-filled syringe and jumped back, lifting my arms like a criminal at gunpoint. He reached up to the endotracheal tube in his mouth and ripped it out.

"I'm Jeff Sageman and my back is killing me!" he yelled. No one moved. We were dumbfounded and frozen in disbelief.

Only Drysdale remained calm and knew what to do.

"Okay, Jeff, just lie down and we'll take care of you," he said, as he put his hand on Jeff's chest and pushed him to lie flat. I was still standing with my arms up in surrender when the senior resident in thoracics arrived and announced himself.

"Hi. Mike Phoenix. Thoracics. What's up?" he asked Drysdale.

Drysdale summarized the case succinctly. "Nineteen-year-old male fell twenty feet with a glass stab through the back into the heart. Dropped his pressure when I pulled out the glass, then needed pericardiocentesis."

Dr. Phoenix looked at the needle with the blood-filled syringe still piercing and hanging from Jeff's chest. "I'll call the OR," was all he said, and he started to walk backwards towards the phone, still looking directly at Jeff.

Just then Jeff fainted again. Drysdale reached for his neck to check his pulse. Nothing.

"Chris. One more time," he looked at me.

I pulled on the syringe, but no more blood came. I moved the needle in and out, still pulling, but nothing came. As I moved in, the ECG fired. I was piercing the heart itself—too deep. I pulled back but could not suck out any more blood.

Dr. Phoenix was suddenly beside me and pushed me away. He pulled the needle right out of Jeff and squirted all the blood onto the blankets between his legs, then pushed the needle back through Jeff's upper abdomen and banged up against his lowest rib. He angled the needle downwards and slipped it under the rib, pushing the needle to its hub. A foot of metal pierced Jeff's chest. Keeping suction on the syringe, he pulled the needle back slowly. No blood squirted into the barrel.

Without hesitating, he pierced Jeff's body again. Nothing.

"Open the thoracotomy tray," he called, and the nurse rushed to the back shelf. That rarely used tray was at the very bottom.

"We have to crack the chest," he spoke directly to Drysdale. "He won't make it to the OR."

Drysdale moved to the head of the gurney and Phoenix moved to the left side of the bed. While Phoenix put on gloves and poured iodine on Jeff's chest, Drysdale intubated him again. Phoenix took a scalpel and cut deeply between Jeff's left fifth and sixth ribs; the incision curved around his chest from below his nipple towards his side. He then pushed his hand in between the ribs and inserted a rib spreader—two flat metal blades with a crank that allows them to be ratcheted apart. Phoenix turned the ratchet, and the blades clicked apart. He turned the lever as hard as he could, and I thought his ribs would break.

Phoenix then pushed Jeff's lung away with his left hand. There was no way to see inside the deep hole in Jeff's chest, so Phoenix used his fingertips to feel for the heart. When he found it, he reached for the scalpel with his right hand and it completely disappeared into the hole. Phoenix cut a window in the pericardium to relieve the tamponade on the heart.

"Okay," he said as if the problem was solved, but Jeff remained motionless.

"No pulse," Drysdale said from the head of the bed with his fingers on Jeff's neck.

"Let the heart fill," Phoenix responded.

"No pulse," Drysdale returned, not waiting very long. Jeff was dying again.

Phoenix reached back into Jeff's chest and held his heart in his left hand. He squeezed his fingers towards his palm and rhythmically squished Jeff's heart. Open cardiac massage—I had never seen this before.

"I need to call the OR." Phoenix looked at me. "Squeeze his heart."

From the sublime to the ridiculous. Phoenix needed to call the operating room but could not reach the phone because his hand was holding Jeff's heart.

He looked at me to squeeze Jeff's heart.

I moved behind Dr. Phoenix and waited for his instructions. He just pulled his hand out and walked away. No instructions.

I pushed my gloved left hand through the tight space between Jeff's ribs and it popped inside. His ribs squeezed my forearm and I could feel his heart like a chicken breast. I reached around it and pressed it against my palm. It refilled as I let go. I squeezed again and it refilled. This was working.

"Good compressions," Drysdale reported with his finger on Jeff's carotid.

Emboldened, I squeezed harder. Each time Jeff's heart refilled with blood and swelled larger, moving more blood forwards through his aorta and around his body.

Suddenly, I had a horrible thought—what if I put my fingers through his heart? I squeezed more gently and looked up at Drysdale.

He nodded reassuringly. "Good compressions." I think he knew what I was thinking.

Then I felt Jeff's heart come alive. It started to beat inside my hand. I held still and felt it move with a twisting power, beating on its own. I had flushed enough oxygenated blood through to feed his heart and get it started again.

I left my hand in place, scared any movement would undo the current situation. I looked at Dr. Drysdale and told him, "I've stopped but he's going," and waited for instruction.

He said, "Out."

I pulled my hand out.

Drysdale said, "Good pulse," and covered the gaping chest wound with a wet green towel.

Dr. Phoenix returned and reported, "Okay, the OR is ready. We're taking him." With that the orderlies wheeled Jeff Sageman away to the operating room. He was surrounded by a phalanx of nurses scuttling sideways with the stretcher and a respiratory therapist rhythmically squeezing the bag blowing air into his lungs.

I looked at Phoenix and called out to him, "Will he be okay?"

Phoenix looked at me and changed my life forever. "Yeah, he just has a hole in his heart."

The surgeons would suture the hole in Jeff's heart, and he would leave hospital eleven days later. No prescriptions, no ruminations, no arguments. Just problem solved.

My cup of tea.

There was no team debrief. The charge nurse simply handed me another chart. I have no idea who that next patient was or what their problem was. All I could think about was getting home and telling Karla about the drama of my day. This was the most exciting hour of my life. This was the most rewarding hour of my life. This was how I wanted to spend the rest of my life.

———

Jeff's "resurrection" felt like a turning point in my medical career. I suddenly knew with certainty that surgery was the correct pathway for me. I wanted to be the one, like Dr. Phoenix, who could definitively solve the problem. The emergency room was exciting, but this patient's injuries were too complex for them to correct. I wanted to be the person who had enough knowledge and skill to calmly take the patient to the operating room and save them. It was one thing to think about surgery as a possible vocation; it was quite another thing to literally feel it in your own hands. The brief surgery that allowed me to massage Jeff's heart was the most exhilarating thing I had ever experienced, and it gave me a sense of purpose. Earlier in the week I was lost and unsure of my future, but now I knew for sure what to do. This wasn't a matter of logic—it was more like an awakening. *I once was lost but now am found, was blind but now I see.* I was a scientist but the realization felt like a spiritual epiphany. A matter of faith, of having faith.

I trusted I was on the path towards surgery, but the final fork in the road towards neurosurgery was still a ways off. After my internship, I left for Oxford to study the science of the brain for three years, with the hope that this doctoral degree would give me the tools to undertake medical research in the future. During my time at Oxford, the final confirmation that neurosurgery was the right choice for my life would come in a moment of intense personal pain.

3.

BABY MICHAEL

M y memories of living and studying in Oxford have improved over time. Most graduate students filled their days with an eclectic mix of culture, socializing and travel, but I just worked in the lab. In my spare time, I trained as a springboard diver—my athletic passion. In hindsight, I wish I had taken the time to broaden my education, but I was too focused on hurrying to the finish line—namely, a PhD in the Department of Human Anatomy. At Oxford, it's called a DPhil, but both abbreviations stand for the same thing: Doctor of Philosophy.

I do have some fond memories of the city of dreaming spires. At lunchtime on Wednesdays, I played "real tennis" with my supervisor, Professor Charlton, and two of his friends. This medieval racquet sport, the precursor to modern tennis, was popularized in England by Henry VIII. In fact, he was playing a game in Hampton Court when his second wife, Anne Boleyn, was executed. The word "real" comes from the Anglo-French for "royal."

Leaving the lab with its state-of-the-art equipment in 1989, we'd walk down South Parks Road past Rhodes House (1926), Trinity College (1555) and into Merton College (1264). The real tennis court, built in 1595, was designed to resemble a medieval street with sloping walls, a stone floor and galleries that are in play. Learning how to score was harder than hitting the rock-hard balls with our wooden racquets.

I had roots in England—my father was born there and had studied sciences at Trinity in Oxford, then moved to the West Indies ostensibly because there were no teaching jobs in the United Kingdom. He worked as a biology teacher at Harrison College, Barbados. At the time, my mother was a journalist who wrote travel articles for Trans-Canada Airlines. She'd visited Barbados to write an article for the airline's magazine, and that's how they met and married. I was born in Barbados and grew up with a strong Bajan accent. Apparently I spent much of my early childhood in the sea or up a tree. We eventually moved to Canada because the cost of living was too high in Barbados for a teacher to support a family.

I grew up in Port Hope, a small town on the shore of Lake Ontario. The nearest university was in Toronto and my studies began at Trinity College. It was there that I met my sweet wife, Karla. I was playing soccer on the back field and twisted my ankle. My best friend, Paul, was helping me off the field and asked where I wanted to sit down. I looked up and saw Karla sitting with her back against the wall, reading a textbook in the sunshine. "Right beside her," I instructed, and Paul smiled. That was the best decision of my life, and Paul was the best man at our wedding.

By the time I was completing my PhD at Oxford, Karla and I were married and expecting our first child. We flew back to Toronto for Michael's birth, naively scheduling two weeks for the round trip.

The labour was induced, the delivery difficult. The forceps failed, an emergency Caesarean section was needed. Karla was resting on the delivery ward when the nurse told me I was needed urgently in the nursery.

This can't be good, I thought to myself as I slipped out of the room while Karla slept. Walking down the hallway towards the nursery, I was met by an ashen-coloured OB-GYN resident who shocked me into attention.

"Baby Michael has a head injury," she blurted out. "Neurosurgery are on their way!"

The details of the next twenty-four hours are not all clear to me. The stress hormone cortisol can enhance and degrade memories. I remember some moments vividly but others are gone, perhaps suppressed.

Now, thirty years later, I still have difficulty talking about this. Baby Michael's skull had been fractured by the forceps, and he was rushed from the Wellesley Hospital to the Hospital for Sick Children for a CT scan in the middle of the night. I followed and watched the images of the CT scan scrolling out, unbearably slowly, one at a time on the monitor. I was waiting to see if there was bleeding in his brain.

None. Just a depressed skull fracture. Of course, only a neurosurgeon could think it was *just* a skull fracture. But by this time, I knew the brain was a jewel inside a jewellery box, the skull. The jewellery box had been broken but the jewel was intact.

I tried to calm myself. Karla was growing desperate—this was a new mother's nightmare. She had not seen the baby after the birth and had woken to the news that he had been taken to the children's hospital in another part of the city.

The following morning, less than a day old, Baby Michael was facing surgery to elevate his skull fracture off his brain and put it back into place. Dr. E. Bruce Hendrick was Canada's first full-time pediatric neurosurgeon. When I met him, he was a big man with meaty hands and a fatherly smile that radiated confidence. I fell under his calming spell. He asked me to wait in his office while he did the surgery. Not a waiting room, but his actual office. This was very unusual, but he knew I had finished medical school in Toronto and was interested in surgery. I sat there alone, looking at all his pictures. He had two kids; one was also named Michael.

Ninety minutes later he returned, still wearing his green scrubs. "Everything went just fine," he reported, and went over the operation as if I was a trusted colleague. By this time, I had not yet begun any neurosurgical training. He overestimated my knowledge but he pulled me up to his.

I was surprised by how much time he spent with me that day. Listening to the old master recount the operation, one that he must have done hundreds of times, I was not only immensely relieved by the positive outcome but captivated by Dr. Hendrick's joy. He was sixty-five years old, and my son would be one of his last cases. It was evident that he was passionate about his work and an excellent teacher. I can still remember every nuance of the operation he described.

When he finished talking to me, he picked up his office phone to call Karla. It took a while to go through the various phone operators, up to the delivery floor, and finally to her bedside. I could hear Karla crying on the other end as Dr. Hendrick explained the good news.

"You are very lucky," he continued.

"How am I lucky?" she asked quietly.

"You will get to take your baby home."

There were three other children in Baby Michael's ward room. One had a brain tumour the size of a baseball in his newborn head. Another was paralyzed from a spinal cord defect. The third had a devastating brain injury, probably from abuse. This was a sad place, but the nurses were heroic. They comforted the tiny patients and their parents and provided surrogate love for the abused child, whose parents I never saw. Pediatric brain surgery seemed to me like it would be too emotionally tough to enjoy. There must be victories, like Baby Michael, but there were far more losses.

A few days later, I brought Michael back to Karla, and our young family was reunited. It was a daunting introduction to parenthood, but we had weathered the storm.

We were thrilled and so very thankful to have our baby with us, healthy and happy. And of course, we remain forever grateful to Dr. Hendrick. Just as Jeff had determined my focus on surgery, so Dr. Hendrick cemented my decision for neurosurgery. But Dr. Hendrick would not have been able to save my son's life—and neurosurgery would not exist—but for the pioneering efforts of courageous surgeons before him. Their story is part of mine. Very briefly, I'd like to share some of the background of how brain surgery has evolved.

4.

A BRIEF HISTORY
OF BRAIN SURGERY

Modern brain surgery is a recent development in the story of medicine; it is barely a hundred years old. The human brain was long considered to be too precious to touch, so it required someone who was scientifically curious, surgically trained, and perhaps emotionally blunted to the consequence of failure to attempt surgery on the brain.

While there is some dispute as to whether Europe or North America produced the world's first neurosurgeon, there is evidence that significant cranial procedures were undertaken in ancient times in Africa, India and South America.

In January 1862, a Connecticut-born antiquities dealer and amateur Egyptologist, Edwin Smith—who lived much of his adult life in Egypt—bought a papyrus document from a local dealer named Mustafa Agha. This hand-printed scroll, on a paper-like substance made from the papyrus plant, most likely originated from the necropolis in Thebes. Smith was never able to adequately translate the hieroglyphs and, after his death, the scroll was donated by his daughter to the New York Historical Society. Translated and published in 1930, its contents caused a worldwide sensation.

Unknowingly, Smith had acquired the oldest medical text ever written, dated to approximately 1600 BCE. Experts have determined it is a copy of a much older surgical treatise from around 3500 BCE, and it remains the earliest known text to offer practical medical treatments for patients rather than attempts at magic or quackery. It describes forty-eight medical cases; the first twenty-seven are concerned with head injuries. Case number 6 mentions a scalp wound with a skull fracture beneath it and "something oozing out." Looking into a gaping scalp wound, the author found a pulsating structure with corrugated edges. This is the first known description of the human brain.

There are six other cases dealing with injuries to the throat and neck; two concerned with the clavicle; twelve regarding injuries to the sternum, shoulders or humerus (the long bone from the shoulder to the elbow); and the incomplete forty-eighth case deals with the spine. Some of the advice, including directives on when not to bother treating a patient with a lethal injury, could have been written as recently as the 1800s. Although cases concerning head injuries dominate, the Egyptians did not operate on the brain, which they did not consider particularly important. When they embalmed bodies, they pulled the brain out through the nose with a long, sharp hook and discarded it.

Only the heart was left in the body, as it was thought to be the centre of a person's being and intelligence. The argument over whether the heart or brain was the source of thought would be solved by Leonardo da Vinci's experiments on frogs in the late fifteenth century. He wrote that a frog died instantly when its brainstem was pithed but lingered after its heart was removed.

Egyptologists like to suggest the Edwin Smith Papyrus could have been written by the renowned pyramid architect Imhotep, chancellor to the pharaoh Djoser, although there is no evidence that he was a physician. I first heard about it in a medical school lecture on spinal injuries, and it was exhibited for the public at the Metropolitan Museum of Art in New York in 2005–2006, coincidental with a new translation. The papyrus's historical significance was magnified to me and, no doubt, to many others by the fact that it was translated into English and displayed in New York. It's hard to imagine how many other remarkable medical documents have been ignored by Western-biased medical training programs because they were not translated into English. We may now marvel at New Age medicine, which promotes a healthy balance in life and teaches how to prevent illness rather than how to treat it, but Eastern physicians have been practising this way for a thousand years.

While researching this book, I discovered several Indian physicians who never appeared in any of my training. The stories of their extraordinary achievements are buried in esoteric journals and, if not for my Indian colleagues, would remain unknown to me. One such physician was Susruta, who lived probably before 600 BCE and wrote a surgical treatise called the *Susruta Samhita*. In it he described three hundred operations, including procedures dealing with penetrating injuries to the skull. Another was Jivaka, the personal physician to the Buddha, who lived in the fifth century BCE. He was also reputed to have performed complex procedures, including once opening the skull to remove a tumour.

There is clear, irrefutable evidence of early brain surgery in South America. The Inca controlled a vast area of the Andean region of South America around 1500 CE, and numerous skulls have been found from that era with holes made in them, the result of a surgical procedure call trepanation. It is still a common surgery today—former president Jimmy Carter had it in 2019, and football player Diego

Maradona had it in 2020. Neurosurgeons use the hole in the skull to remove a blood clot and take the pressure off the brain.

What is remarkable is that 80 percent of these trepanned skulls show evidence that the patient survived. New bone growth around the site of the trepanning could only have occurred if the patient had lived. The rate of survival was shockingly good when you compare the survival rate of similar operations during the American Civil War some four hundred years later, which was only 50 percent. We do not know why the Inca used trepanation, but they were clearly skilled at it.

A 2018 study in *World Neurosurgery* of trepanned skulls from pre-Columbian Peru showed an improvement in survival rates over time. Beginning in 400 BCE, approximately 40 percent of patients survived. Improvements in instruments and techniques increased the survival rate to 53 percent by 1000–1400 CE and to 80 percent at the height of the Inca empire a hundred years later.

Many of these skulls had additional evidence of trauma, such as fractures, so we can assume that these trepanations were a form of treatment for the injuries. The Inca used a semicircular knife, a *tumi*, to cut through the skull. I still do at least one of these operations every week using a high-speed drill. However, some of the Inca skulls had no evidence of trauma, which suggests that trepanation was also used for other reasons. The Inca did not have a written language, so we can only guess what the other conditions might have been—possibly headaches?

Trepanned skulls have been found throughout the world, but the ones in Peru have benefited from the dry climate of the high Andes and are thus the best preserved and most studied as the oldest surviving evidence of surgery. The Inca skulls also have examples with multiple holes and holes replaced with gold.

In one site in France, a third of the Neolithic skulls (6500 BCE) had trepanation. There are no trepanned skulls before the Neolithic period, or New Stone Age, perhaps because without a sophisticated stone tool, it would be very difficult to cut through a skull. About 10 percent of Neolithic skulls have holes bored into them, and a few even suggest that the patient or victim survived.

But surgery on the skull is not brain surgery, it is more cranial orthopaedics. The skull is after all just another bone. I explain this to my patients (and orthopaedic friends) with my favourite analogy—the skull is just the jewellery box, not the jewel.

The first recorded operation to remove an intracranial tumour (one inside the skull) took place in Glasgow in 1879. Born and raised in Scotland, William Macewen was a general surgeon at the Glasgow Royal Infirmary. We know that three years before this first brain surgery, he had recommended the procedure for a brain abscess in a young boy named John McKinley, but the parents had refused. After the boy died, an autopsy confirmed the abscess was where Macewen had predicted.

In Macewen's iconic address to the British Medical Association in 1888, he said there were two factors that had led to the possibility of successful brain surgery. First was the development of aseptic surgery, meaning free from contamination by harmful bacteria. Macewen had been a student of the Quaker Joseph Lister in Glasgow, who pioneered aseptic surgery by using phenol (carbolic acid) to clean his instruments and wounds. In the 1850s, Louis Pasteur had introduced the concept of microscopic creatures—bacteria—being capable of causing disease, thereby leading Lister to propose that phenol might be used to kill germs and prevent infections arising from surgeries.

Macewen was once visited by an American surgeon who was keen to learn about this new business of cleanliness during surgery. The American asked Macewen if he should bathe before surgery, and the doctor replied, with his acerbic Scottish wit, "In Scotland, we bathe whether we operate or not."

The second factor Macewen revealed was the new science of neurology and its ability to localize a lesion within the brain based on the defects it caused in the patient. If a patient had seizures in their left arm, there was a predictable lesion in their right frontal lobe. Even if a patient's scalp and skull looked normal, neurologists could confidently predict that there would be a lesion beneath it.

The combination of these two advances—together with the recently discovered implementation of anaesthesia—enabled Macewen to be the first to successfully remove a tumour from inside the skull. (The word "tumour" is taken from the Latin word for a mass or swelling and does not necessarily refer to a cancer.)

The tumour of Macewen's patient may have been a tuberculoma, but no pathology was ever reported. A tuberculoma is a mass or tumour of connective tissue triggered by an infection from the tuberculosis bacilli. Tuberculosis, or TB, was prevalent in Glasgow at the time. The patient was a fourteen-year-old girl, who recovered quickly and was said to be "fully employable a few months later." This was, after all, 1879.

Macewen was also an accomplished self-promoter who published the case report in the *Glasgow Medical Journal* before his young patient had even left the hospital. The "father of neurosurgery" was a man who had a great deal to boast about. As early as 1880 he started a training program for nurses that stressed aseptic practices. He was knighted in 1902. In response to the plethora of returning military men who had lost their limbs during the First World War, he founded the Princess Louise Scottish Hospital for Limbless Sailors and Soldiers in 1916 near Glasgow (now the Erskine Hospital). Here he collaborated with engineers and workers at the nearby shipyards to implement the groundbreaking manufacture of artificial limbs.

In 1883—just four years after Macewen's first tumour extraction— Francesco Durante at the Royal University (now "La Sapienza") in

Rome performed a similar operation. Durante's patient was a thirty-five-year-old woman who had a tumour the size of an apple removed from the floor of her skull behind her eye. She lived for many years after the surgery.

Durante was a young Italian surgeon who not only boasted an even bigger beard than Macewen, but was also a friend of the Austro-Hungarian emperor, Franz Joseph, and operated on one of his daughters. His reward for success was two white stallions from the famous Spanish Stable.

Durante correctly predicted that "the cranial cavity may, in future, justly enter into the dominion of surgery." It's important to note that both these operations performed by Macewen and Durante involved tumours located inside the skull but outside the brain.

The first "successful" removal of a tumour within the brain itself was undertaken on November 25, 1884, by (Lord) Joseph Lister's nephew, Mr. Rickman Godlee. In the United Kingdom, physicians are bestowed with the title "doctor" when they graduate from medical school, but those who complete their surgical training are called Mr. (not Dr.) to distinguish them from their medical colleagues. Mr. Godlee was a thirty-five-year-old junior surgeon working in London. His patient was a twenty-five-year-old Scottish farmer who had developed daily seizures on the left side of his body.

As his condition worsened, he became paralyzed on his left side and developed excruciating headaches. As was recorded in an 1885 medical article by neurologist Alexander Hughes Bennett:

> The terrible sufferings of the patient rendered life intolerable to him. All remedial measures having failed, and as it was obvious that his symptoms were extending, and that a fatal termination was not far distant, it was determined that

an attempt be made to remove the morbid lesion. It was hoped that even if such a proceeding was not permanently successful it might alleviate some of the more pressing symptoms. The novelty and risks of the proposed treatment having been fully placed before the patient and his friends, they readily consented to the adoption of any measures which offered any prospects of mitigating the urgent distress or of averting a certain death.

Godlee explored inside the right side of the patient's brain near the posterior portion of his frontal lobe. The right side of the brain was known to control the left side of the body, and the part of the brain responsible for movement was the posterior frontal lobe. The surgery took two hours while the patient was under chloroform anaesthesia. A tumour the size of a "pigeon's egg" was removed completely, and the patient recovered.

But Mr. Godlee was missing three things that modern neurosurgeons take for granted: antibiotics (accidentally discovered by Alexander Fleming in 1928), cautery to stop bleeding (developed by William Bovie and Harvey Cushing in 1926), and a microscope to see exactly what they are doing (popularized by Gazi Yaşargil in the 1960s).

Among the important visitors observing this unprecedented operation (in what is known in England as the operating theatre) was twenty-seven-year-old Victor Horsley, who was inspired to become the world's first neurosurgeon. Also present were three of the leading neurologists of their era—Drs. Alexander Hughes Bennett, John Hughlings Jackson, and David Ferrier—who collectively pioneered the science of estimating where in the brain a problem occurred by the altered functions it caused. They wanted to see if their new science of "cerebral localization" could be applied in practice.

The patient did well initially. An unsigned report of the case quickly appeared as an editorial in the *Lancet* in 1884. Unfortunately, on the fourth day, when his dressings were changed, they were clearly infected. The patient's course went from bad to worse, and he died twenty-eight days after the operation. When an autopsy was performed on Christmas Eve, the pathologist triumphantly announced that no residual tumour was found. This may have been the origin of the terrible phrase, "The operation was successful, but the patient died."

Godlee would never operate on the brain again.

In their 1885 paper in the *British Medical Journal* describing the case, Hughes Bennett and Godlee prophetically stated:

> In conclusion, we would observe that, although unfortunate in this instance life was not permanently preserved, the experience gained by the case leads us to believe that there is an encouraging prospect for the future of cerebral medicine and surgery, and that as a tumor of the brain can be diagnosed with precision and successfully removed without immediate danger to life.

While the neurologists involved in the case were very pleased, the public was not. There was an outcry in the *Times* following the sensational publication of the case. Over the ensuing three months, no less than sixty-four letters to the editor argued vehemently for or against this work. Antivivisectionists, for example, were angry that scientists had experimented upon stray dogs to learn the function of different parts of the brain by damaging an area and examining the effects. The scientists' patronizing rebuttal was that it would all be worth it in the end.

All of the physicians who first ventured inside the skull were general surgeons who operated anywhere in the body but very, very rarely inside the head. They removed appendixes, set broken bones and incised any abscesses. They were reluctant explorers, spurred on by the certain fatality of brain tumours and infections.

———

Perhaps the most famous patient with a brain abscess was King Henry II of France. The story of his jousting injury on June 30, 1559, and his subsequent treatments by Ambroise Paré and Andreas Vesalius is recounted in wonderful detail in Sam Kean's book *The Tale of the Dueling Neurosurgeons*.

Although neither of these physicians were neurosurgeons, the story is compelling. Paré was the most famous surgeon of his day, and Vesalius produced the most exquisite anatomy text ever published. The king had been pierced through his left eye and temple by the lance of his young opponent. Unfortunately, the combined talents of these giants of medieval medicine could not save the king, particularly as this was the era before Macewen had popularized aseptic procedures. The king died an agonizing death ten days later. No one benefited from that encounter, with the possible exception of Nostradamus.

Nostradamus was a French physician who became famous for being able to predict the future. In *Les Prophéties*, he wrote poetic quatrains about the future. The book, published in 1555, four years before the king's death, included the prophetic lines:

> *The young lion will overcome the older one,*
> *On the field of combat in single battle;*
> *He will pierce his eyes through a golden cage,*
> *Two wounds made one, then he dies a cruel death.*

I had a very similar encounter with a non-royal but no less noble patient, Robert Charles. A small, soft-spoken Indigenous man who wore his grey hair long in a ponytail, he was walking through the Downtown Eastside of Vancouver one day when he felt someone punch him in the eye. He was startled for a moment and did not see who had hit him. He sat down on a bench to collect his thoughts, then continued on his way.

When his senses cleared, Robert noticed that he had double vision—he saw two images of the people walking towards him along Hastings Street. He decided to walk over to the emergency department at St. Paul's Hospital to get checked out. An emergency physician confirmed that Robert was seeing double, and a CT scan was performed to see if there was any damage to his eye.

The scan revealed a frightening truth. There was a paintbrush jammed in beside his left eye (causing the double vision), and the deep end was stuck through the roof of his eye socket into his brain. The handle of the brush had broken off and was concealed by his eyelid. The metal end, which held the horsehair fibres of the brush, had entered the lower left side of his brain and then crossed the midline to lodge in his right thalamus.

I was called by the emergency doctor with the memorable opening line, "You're not going to believe this, but . . ."

We brought Robert to the operating room minutes later. I was ready to open his skull and deal with any bleeding. After he was anaesthetized, I lifted up his eyelid and used a clamp to grab the protruding wooden end of the brush. I slowly pulled seven inches of paintbrush out of his brain. A stat CT scan showed no bleeding or retained pieces.

I had one advantage over the combined talents of Paré and Vesalius—antibiotics.

The following day, Robert took his antibiotics and walked out of the hospital (against my advice). I wrote the case up in a 2005 paper entitled "Artistic Assault: An Unusual Penetrating Head Injury Reported as a Trivial Facial Trauma." I stayed in contact with Robert as long as he would let me. But he had neither a phone nor a home, so it was difficult to keep in touch or book an appointment.

On rare occasions, and without notice, Robert would drop by the office when he was walking near Vancouver General. He remained quietly dignified and hadn't sought out his assailant or contacted the authorities to report the assault. He was not angry when I first told him about the paintbrush. He had met adversity before, he would surely meet it again. He was at peace with his place in the world.

The paintbrush, encased in acrylic, sits on my desk.

To return to the history of neurosurgery, the evolution from a general surgeon operating on the skull to a neurosurgeon operating inside the brain came in February 1886 with the emergence of Mr. Victor Horsley.

At the National Hospital for the Paralyzed and Epileptic in Queen Square, London, neurologists had pioneered the ability to localize a lesion within the brain—even if it made no observable changes to the head or skull. By studying patients with epilepsy and paralysis, they were able to correlate the symptoms in life with the pathology after death. They were now ready to remove brain pathology from their living patients; all they needed was a surgeon willing to do it. After two surgeons at their hospital said no thanks, they hired Horsley.

Victor Horsley was born in Kensington, London, in 1857. Named Victor Alexander by his godmother, Queen Victoria, he lived a life of privilege. His father was a successful painter and his sister a close friend of Felix Mendelssohn. At the time of his appointment as the first neurosurgeon at Queen Square, Horsley was busy with a royal commission to study if Louis Pasteur's claims of a vaccine against rabies were true. And they were.

Within a year, Horsley had completed eleven operations. All of his patients survived, except one. He removed the first spinal cord tumour. He cured an epileptic for the first time by removing the scar tissue caused by a previous brain injury. Among Horsley's many achievements were understanding that the vagus nerve controlled the larynx (voice box), which would become truly relevant to me and my future patients. He also invented bone wax—which would have been immensely helpful in Liberia. Horsley was brilliant but not meticulous. He operated quickly, and his speed made it difficult to learn from him. This may have sown the seeds for the first rivalry in neurosurgery.

My colleagues from the United States will tell you that the world's first "full-time" neurosurgeon was the American Dr. Harvey Cushing, because Horsley continued to operate on the thyroid gland in the neck during his career as a neurosurgeon (a skill that would also have been helpful in Liberia). Cushing had impeccable training as an undergraduate at Yale, a medical student at Harvard, and a resident at Johns Hopkins, where he met William Osler, the most respected physician of the time. Cushing would write the definitive double-volume biography of Sir William Osler in 1925 and receive the Pulitzer Prize for his work. In a cruel twist of fate, Osler's only son, Revere, died in Cushing's care after the Battle of Ypres in the First World War.

After completing his medical studies, Cushing travelled for four-teen months through Europe visiting the great surgeons and scientists of the day, including Victor Horsley. As much as he admired Osler, Cushing dismissed Horsley. In a biography of Cushing written by the Yale neuroscientist John Fulton, there is a telling passage in which Cushing describes watching Horsley operate:

> Horsley dashed upstairs, had his patient under ether in five minutes, and was operating fifteen minutes after he entered the house; made a great hole in the woman's skull, pushed up the temporal lobe—blood everywhere, gauze packed into the middle fossa, the ganglion cut, the wound closed, and was out of the house less than an hour after he had entered it.

Cushing left London for Baltimore shortly thereafter, reportedly saying there was nothing of modern neurosurgery that he could learn from Horsley. He forged his own path, and all neurosurgeons in North America can trace their training back to him.

Cushing trained Kenneth McKenzie (Canada's first neurosurgeon).

McKenzie trained Frank Turnbull (British Columbia's first neurosurgeon).

Turnbull trained Felix Durity (Vancouver's first neurosurgical resident).

Durity trained me.

I found it hard to call him Felix even after I joined him on staff at Vancouver General Hospital—and I still do, years later. Dr. Durity is an impressive and imposing man. Born and raised in Trinidad, he came to Canada and, after graduating from UBC medical school, became the first neurosurgical resident in the Vancouver program. Black surgeons were a rarity in Canada in the 1970s, but when I met him in the early 1990s, he was just the teacher who knew everything and performed all the hardest operations. I remember assisting him on more than one marathon tumour case and finishing midway through the next day. After finishing a surgery, he would treat himself to a coffee, which he always drank from a Styrofoam bowl designed for soup. Like most of the great neurosurgeons, his stature allowed him to develop eccentricities unfettered by convention. No one was going to tell Felix Durity to drink from a cup.

Cushing and Horsley had their eccentricities too, but they were typically diametrically opposed. Cushing was a slow and methodical surgeon; Horsley was fast and furious. Cushing was a chain smoker; Horsley hated smokers and never drank. Cushing was a surgical workaholic; Horsley had many passions outside medicine. He was active in politics, supported social welfare and championed the suffragette movement. Cushing scoffed at female doctors. Their deaths were also markedly different. Sir Victor Horsley died of heat stroke at age fifty-nine in Syria at a military hospital where he was volunteering during the First World War. Cushing retired to Yale University and died at age seventy of a heart attack while organizing the medical library that bears his name.

Cushing was an excellent artist who, together with his pathologist, Dr. Louise Eisenhardt, described and categorized all the different tumours that could develop within the brain. Looking through the online collection of images in the Cushing Library at Yale, one caught my eye in particular. Pictured here are images of Cushing and Horsley around the time they met in London in 1900. The third image is a drawing by Cushing describing his operative technique to expose the brain. The patient looks remarkably like Horsley!

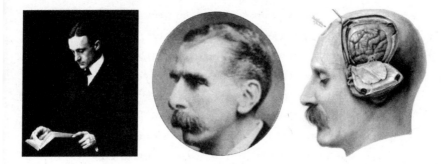

Images of Dr. Harvey Cushing (left) and Mr. Victor Horsley (centre), circa 1900, and a surgical drawing by Cushing (right) demonstrating how to open the scalp and skull to expose the brain.

Cushing discovered and named Cushing's syndrome—a disease caused by a pituitary tumour overproducing the steroid hormone—in 1932. The malady can be cured by removing the tumour—an operation that Cushing pioneered. He also pioneered electric cautery during surgery and clarified the body's response to increased intracranial pressure through experiments on dogs.

Arguably his three daughters, known as "the fabulous Cushing sisters," became more renowned than he was, but for different reasons. Betsey Cushing married the son of then president Franklin Delano Roosevelt, and when Eleanor Roosevelt was away, Betsey hosted dignitaries at the White House. Minnie Cushing (Minnie Astor Fosburgh) married William Vincent Astor, who became the richest man in America after his father, John Jacob Astor IV, died on the *Titanic*. Babe Cushing (Babe Mortimer Paley) became a fashion icon working at *Vogue* magazine. In 1941, *Time* magazine voted her the "second best dressed woman in the world" after Wallis Simpson. Truman Capote quipped, "Babe had only one flaw, she was perfect."

Cushing trained a series of surgeons who went on to popularize neurosurgery around the world, most notably Walter Dandy. Dr. Dandy kept a picture of himself playing tennis with Cushing on his mantelpiece, but Mrs. Dandy instructed her children never to speak about or ask about the other man in the picture. The master and the medical acolyte did not get along.

Dandy grew up in humble circumstances but excelled academically. He was awarded a Rhodes scholarship, which he declined in order to study medicine at Johns Hopkins. He then began surgical training at Hopkins and spent a year in Cushing's laboratory, becoming Cushing's clinical assistant in 1911.

Letters home to his parents portray an ambitious young man daring to outdo his mentor. In one famous case, Cushing had said that surgery for an epileptic sailor was useless, but Dandy performed the technically challenging operation and improved the patient. On another occasion, there were three patients with similar problems. Cushing operated on two of them and both had complications; Dandy did the third flawlessly.

Many patients came to Baltimore just to have the famous Harvey Cushing perform their surgery, but he was often away lecturing and Dandy sometimes convinced the patients to let him do the procedure. In a letter home, he wrote, "I think I will do it in a couple of days rather than wait until he comes back. Gee, won't he be sore to think a young sprout is stealing his thunder."

In 1913, Cushing was invited to lead the surgical department at the newly opened Peter Bent Brigham Hospital in Boston. Dandy was surprised when he did not ask him to come, and devastated when he was told why. Cushing told Dandy that he had "no imagination and should go West where the requirements were not so stringent."

When Cushing went to Boston, Dandy stayed in Baltimore, where he did outstanding research in his laboratory at Johns Hopkins on the production and flow of cerebrospinal fluid. As we've seen, this water-like fluid is produced inside the brain and flows through cavities, called ventricles, and finally out and around the outside of the brain where it is absorbed. It's the fluid that leaks from your ears after a severe head injury cracks open the skull. Leonardo da Vinci was the first to draw the ventricles; Dandy was the first to understand CSF was produced there.

If the flow of this cerebrospinal fluid is blocked, the ventricles will distend with the backed-up fluid and cause a lethal condition called hydrocephalus—like Joshua and Saika in Liberia had. Dandy modelled this effect in dogs and then made two monumental medical advances.

First, he operated on 381 patients with hydrocephalus by either removing the source of cerebrospinal fluid or rerouting its flow. Second, he used air injected into the ventricles to see them on an X-ray.

This was revolutionary. Normally, an X-ray just showed the bone, but now you could see the internal anatomy of the brain. With air trapped inside the ventricles, its outline appeared as a darker shadow on the X-ray. Any tumour, blood clot or abscess inside the brain distorted the contours of the ventricles and could therefore be detected.

The neurologists had been good at localization, but Dandy's ventriculogram was better, allowing neurosurgeons to more accurately localize any unusual growth within the brain. It became widespread around the world—except in Boston, where Cushing did not like the technique—and was only superseded by the CT scan in the 1980s.

In Vancouver, when I began my neurosurgical training in 1990, the ventriculogram was the stuff of legend. Horror stories associated with it were recounted by the elder statesmen of neurosurgery. Dr. Durity told me that there was a special chair the patients would be strapped into for the test. A lumbar puncture was used to inject air through the lower back into the cerebrospinal fluid surrounding the spinal cord, and the patients were then rotated upside down and in all manner of directions to bubble the air up into their ventricles. This would typically cause projectile vomiting and often precipitate unconsciousness due to a potentially lethal distortion of the brain following the sudden pressure changes inside the head.

Patients would be booked for "the chair" at 7 a.m. and for their emergency craniotomy "to follow." Dr. Durity would then race them down the hallway, still strapped in the chair, and burst through the swinging doors into the operating room with the now unconscious patient.

Dandy was nominated for the Nobel Prize in Physiology or Medicine in 1933 for this work, but lost out to Thomas Hunt Morgan "for his discoveries concerning the role played by the chromosome in heredity." Both Horsley and Cushing were also unsuccessful Nobel Prize nominees. The great German neurosurgeon, Otfrid Foerster, was also nominated but would not win. No neurosurgeon has ever won the Nobel Prize except for one—sort of.

Dr. Egas Moniz received the 1949 Nobel Prize for Physiology or Medicine in recognition for inventing the lobotomy, but Moniz was actually a neurologist, not a neurosurgeon. He came from an aristocratic Portuguese family and enjoyed an extraordinary life as a politician and then physician. The story of how he conceived of the lobotomy operation and how neurosurgeons rapidly adopted it, ignored its misuse, and ultimately abandoned it forever is a frightening tale of caution. It's a betrayal the public has not fully recovered from; neurosurgery still suffers under its cloud. More advanced operations—which can treat severe depression—are still illegal in Japan and Oregon because of the continuing backlash against lobotomy.

Dr. Moniz attended the second International Congress of Neurology in London in 1935, where he heard a lecture from John Fulton (the Yale neuroscientist who would later write the Cushing biography that criticized Horsley). Fulton was studying the functions of the frontal lobes in primates. He described two chimpanzees who would get angry or agitated if they made a mistake during a test that had a food reward for correct responses. After he deliberately damaged the chimpanzees' frontal lobes, the animals no longer got "frustrated" when they made mistakes.

When Moniz returned to Lisbon, he convinced his neurosurgical colleague to perform prefrontal leucotomies (cutting the white matter connections to the patients' frontal lobes) on patients with mostly depression or schizophrenia. They completed twenty operations within three months. Moniz reported that one-third of the patients were significantly improved, one-third were better and one-third were unchanged. Importantly, he stated that none had deteriorated after the surgery—though this was not true.

These reported results were an unprecedented improvement in the treatment of mental illness. Almost too good to believe. Until then severely mentally ill patients had had no treatment. Ice bath therapy had failed, insulin coma was dangerous, and doctors sometimes deemed it necessary for certain patients to be locked up away from the public, often in horrific and abusive conditions.

There was some push-back against Moniz's claims from the local psychiatry community at the time, those who knew the patients involved in the surgeries. Dr. Sobral Cid, who referred his own patients to Moniz for the procedure, said they came back to him "diminished." He subsequently denounced the operation publicly.

This did not deter Moniz, who was an influential person and well respected. (He had represented Portugal as foreign minister during the signing of the Treaty of Versailles that ended the First World War.) He was able to popularize the operation ahead of the eventual realization that lobotomy patients paid a terrible price for their reduced complaints of depression and psychosis: many had turned into drooling zombies unable to complain or care.

During the 1930s lobotomy took off in the United States, Italy, France, Brazil, Cuba, the United Kingdom, Scandinavia, Japan, Romania and the USSR. Its popularity may have been boosted by the fact that it made the custodial care of these patients much easier. Some government asylums were emptied of many of their long-term residents, and the resultant economic benefits were not lost on the politicians. Of course, the recognition of this procedure by the Nobel Prize committee helped legitimize its widespread use. Its misuse and abuse were initially overlooked amid the euphoria of finally having a treatment for severe mental illness. The fact that it did not work as reported was also ignored by many medical professionals. Soviet psychiatrists were the first to ban the procedure in 1950 because "through lobotomy an insane person is changed into an idiot." Many countries eventually followed.

The criteria for this surgery was also recklessly vague and discriminatory. Children with behavioural problems, homosexuals, criminals and patients unable to make an informed decision about the procedure were mixed in with those with schizophrenia or depression. A psychiatrist in the United States, William Freeman, whose career is chronicled in a book called *The Lobotomist*, famously drove around the country in his "lobotomobile" performing the procedure with an ice pick.

John F. Kennedy's sister Rosemary had a lobotomy and spent the rest of her life institutionalized. Eva Perón had a lobotomy in secret. Only a post-mortem examination of her skull gave away the diagnosis.

As public sentiment swung strongly against lobotomy, the popular press, initially in favour, began to vilify the procedure. The 1962 novel *One Flew Over the Cuckoo's Nest* by Ken Kesey, and its Oscar-winning movie adaptation, cemented the reputation of lobotomy as an evil operation. All psychiatric surgery, even modern procedures that are known to work, is still banned in one state, Oregon—the state where Kesey lived.

There is no other example in the history of surgery where one operation has risen and fallen in favour quite so profoundly. Neurosurgery seems to attract extremes—both in the operations and the operators. I have only met two people convicted of murder and both were neurosurgeons. Their heinous crimes made national news but one detail about Mohammed Shamji, the Canadian neurosurgeon who killed his wife, was omitted. The day after the crime, he performed several operations flawlessly. A colleague of mine was in the operating room at the time and later phoned me as the saga was unravelling and said, "You're not going to believe this, but . . ."

I want to end this anecdotal history of neurosurgery on a high note, which is easy to do, since I've saved arguably the best for last: one of my heroes, Dr. Wilder Penfield. Born in Spokane, Washington, in 1891, he later became a Canadian citizen and lived most of his life in Montreal. His mother, a teacher separated from his physician father, wanted Wilder to get a Rhodes scholarship and therefore enrolled him in Princeton University: every state got a scholarship, and New Jersey was a small state. He played on Princeton's football team, was a good student and became class president.

My mother, as a CBC reporter in Montreal, interviewed Dr. Penfield. She found him tall, handsome and disarmingly charming, and said that he commanded the room with a calm confidence. Consequently my mother encouraged me to apply for the Rhodes scholarship "like Dr. Penfield"; with that award, I spent my three years at Oxford, studying neurophysiology.

Penfield's own studies of neurophysiology with the Nobel laureate Sir Charles Sherrington at Oxford were interrupted by an injury sustained during the First World War, when his ship returning from France

77

was torpedoed. He recuperated at Sir William Osler's home in Oxford and returned to America to study medicine at Johns Hopkins, eventually doing his surgical internship under Harvey Cushing in Boston.

He began his career as a neurosurgeon in New York. There he met the billionaire David Rockefeller, who wanted to endow an institute for Penfield to study the surgical treatment of epilepsy. After Penfield moved to Montreal to become the first neurosurgeon at McGill University, the Rockefeller funding followed him. He founded the Montreal Neurological Institute, which became the mecca for the surgical treatment of epilepsy.

Among the surgeon's legacies are the discoveries he made using local anaesthesia for brain surgery, a procedure he learned from the German neurosurgeon Otfrid Foerster in 1927. Once the scalp was anaesthetized, surgery could be performed through the skull and into the brain, because those structures have no pain sensation. My patient Robert Charles, when he was stabbed by a paintbrush, only complained of a sore eye.

Using this method, Penfield electrically stimulated the exposed brain of his awake patients to test the function of each part. He found that discrete areas controlled specific muscles on the opposite side of the body, and when he mapped out these areas on the brain's frontal cortex, they formed a little human body—a homunculus. When he stimulated the temporal lobe, he could trigger memories and the sensation of déjà vu. A Google doodle on January 26, 2018, honoured the moment when Penfield stimulated a patient's brain and she said, "I smell burnt toast."

Penfield's portrait still hangs in Rhodes House at the University of Oxford. His ashes are buried beside his wife's on the family farm near Lake Memphrémagog, Quebec, which was bought with funds he received from the German government as compensation for the injuries he'd sustained during the First World War. I have admired Penfield since reading his autobiography, *No Man Alone: A Neurosurgeon's Life*, as a teenager at my mother's encouragement. He moved to Canada and discovered fundamental truths about the brain and its function, but also learned as much as he could from each of his patients.

Neurosurgery has continued to make advances over the decades. The rate of mortality following brain tumour surgery has dropped steadily from 37 percent in 1920 to just over 1 percent at the present time. In the United States, mortality is still twice as high for Medicaid patients as for those with private insurance, but that societal discrepancy is a problem not unique to neurosurgery.

The psychological stress on a surgeon who lost a third of their patients must have been crushing. The earliest neurosurgeons were often described as bold or brave, but the truth is they were not risking their own lives, they were risking others', and a sociopath was better able to weather the storms of repeated failure than their empathetic colleagues.

Neurosurgeons of the late twentieth century were notorious for their poor manners and eccentricities. Dandy threw instruments at his nurses. Cushing was feared by everyone (even Dandy). Gazi Yaşargil, head of neurosurgery at the University of Zurich, only ever allowed one nurse to assist him—his wife, Dianne. Yaşargil, who has been given the moniker "father of modern neurosurgery," is credited with popularizing the operating microscope, which allows neurosurgeons to see exactly what they are doing. It was a monumental advance for the field.

Why did (do?) so many pre-eminent neurosurgeons yell at their nurses? Is it the stress of the job? Does a high-pressure type of job just attract a mercurial person? One interesting suggestion came from a colleague of mine who is notorious for this particular offence. When a surgeon makes a mistake during an operation, it can paralyze them with all the thoughts of what might happen or need to be done. If they immediately blame someone, their nurse, for example, they can refocus their attention on fixing the mistake that is that person's, not their own. They are not emotionally distracted by a sense of culpability in that moment.

Although the neurosurgeon's temperament may not have improved over the years, technological advances have continually improved our outcomes. Platinum electrodes can now be accurately placed deep within the brain and connected to pacemakers that can stimulate the brain into better functioning. This technology of deep brain stimulation has helped over 200,000 patients with Parkinson's disease. Our team was the first to use it to improve the voice of patients with spasmodic dysphonia—a disorder of speech that makes communication difficult.

Advances in imaging have allowed us to see smaller objects, and when you are operating, seeing is everything. Computers have allowed virtual planning of operations; the combination of these two technologies has allowed computer-assisted guidance to the operative target. Of course, it still requires a surgeon to get there.

5.

EMILY & LEO

The stories of the next two patients are inextricably intertwined. Emily was the first patient in the world to be diagnosed and surgically cured of HELPS (hemi-laryngopharyngeal spasm); Leo was the second. They were both my patients. And the anatomical source of their choking and coughing affliction wouldn't have been discovered if they hadn't fought the medical system to be understood and recognized.

Their personal descriptions of their symptoms and their cure following my surgery proved that HELPS was a real medical disease with a real treatment.

Both Emily and Leo were repeatedly told by their doctors that their problems were "all in their head." No one believed them because their unique constellation of symptoms had never been attributed to a specific medical condition. I will outline how this medical bewilderment affected their lives and how, eventually, we uncovered the cause of their suffering. I've recounted their plights as best I can.

Emily, in particular, refused to be ignored and never gave up hope that she would be understood. Her courage and tenacity were an inspiration to me. She forced me to look beyond my medical training and consider the possibility of a completely new disease.

EMILY

When Emily Murphy was being wheeled on a gurney into the trauma bay at the small Peace Arch Hospital, the forty-six-year-old florist squeezed out the same words that would be universally recognized six years later as the rallying cry for Black Lives Matter.

"I can't breathe."

Three people heard her, and each had a different reaction.

Arthur had seen Emily, his wife, choke before, but never to this extent. He felt desperate, helpless—and shamefully glad. The couple had visited this emergency room several times, but each time the problem had resolved itself spontaneously, leaving them both feeling sheepish. No one had ever explained what had happened, or why, or whether it would ever happen again. They had just been discharged with a dismissive "Well, you're fine now."

During their last visit, three weeks earlier, Arthur had felt the staff thought they should not have come in at all. The emergency doctor had asked if Emily had a psychiatric history, implying the symptoms might be attributable to a mental health issue. Now Arthur worried the doctors might again be wondering if Emily was somehow making up her symptoms, as if her fear and choking were all a contrivance.

Despite the terrifying situation, this time Arthur was secretly somewhat pleased that Emily's symptoms were much worse. This time the doctors *had* to see how serious her symptoms were—and that could only be a good thing. How else would they ever be able to understand why Emily was repeatedly choking for no reason?

"I can't breathe."

The paramedic wheeling the head of the gurney heard her too. But he was not particularly distressed. His responsibilities were nearly done: his shift would be over in a few minutes at 7 p.m. He would park the gurney in Bay 1, transfer the patient to a stretcher, give a sign-off to the charge nurse, then be on his way. The formal transfer of information from one healthcare worker to another was deliberately quick and dispassionate.

"This forty-six-year-old female presents with choking. She is 'satting' 96 percent on room air, BP is 140 on 85, heart rate is 135, and respirations are hard to tell with her coughing. There's a history of allergies to paints and fumes but not to any meds. Otherwise healthy."

Emily remained sitting upright on the gurney the whole time, clutching at her throat in the universal sign of someone choking. The other paramedic had not heard her. The two paramedics made eye contact and wordlessly choreographed the transfer of the patient onto the waiting stretcher with practised aplomb.

"I can't breathe."

Fortunately, the charge nurse, Maureen Carter, who received the sign-off, had heard Emily's plaintive words. It was that phrase that made her direct Emily to the trauma bay and its one stretcher reserved for serious conditions, mostly heart attacks and car accidents.

It is the charge nurse who is responsible for triaging patients—rapidly assessing their problems and determining if they need to be seen quickly or "in due course." Emily would be seen immediately: the management of an airway problem supersedes all other medical emergencies, even exsanguination (severe loss of blood).

If air is not getting to the lungs, all else fails. If not replenished, the oxygen in a struggling patient's blood is exhausted within a few minutes. Organs that require a lot of energy to function, such as the heart and brain, soon stop working and begin to die. Without the energy from oxygen, the heart cells cannot contract and the heart rate slows to a stop. Blood flow around the body ceases with the last heartbeat.

When the brain's neurons do not have the energy to fire, the complex pattern of brain activity underpinning consciousness fails. Those neurons do not "slip" into unconsciousness—they fall. Within four minutes, the brain cells do not have enough energy to maintain their cellular integrity and begin to die. Permanent brain injury follows, rapidly, relentlessly and irrevocably. Patients deprived of oxygen who somehow manage to survive often spend the rest of their lives in long-term care institutions because they can no longer look after themselves. In the worse-case scenario, often seen as worse than death, the brain has no meaningful function—what scientists call a persistent vegetative state and the lay press cruelly call a "vegetable."

Maureen was an experienced nurse. She had worked for years in the Big House, Vancouver General Hospital, in the intensive care and emergency departments. She could have been a head nurse there but had instead chosen to stay closer to home and avoid a long commute.

An experienced nurse is every patient's greatest asset. In the emergency room, they can be far more important than the doctor. They choose when the patient will be examined, they set the tone of urgency; they give the medications, provide comfort, organize the discharge. They spend more time with the patient. The new medical school curriculum pays lip service to the concept of a well-rounded doctor who understands the patient's emotional and physical needs, but in reality, especially at night in a small emergency room, the doctors are more focused on diagnostic efficiency and treating the symptom rather than the patient.

Maureen absorbed the whole picture, subconsciously comparing Emily to several thousand other patients she had nursed over the last twenty-three years. She knew this was serious but not yet urgent. If Emily could say the words "I can't breathe," she was still able to—to some degree. Patients with complete airway obstruction cannot talk.

Emily's blood oxygen saturation (sats) was 96 percent. This was normal. The paramedic had made clear her vitals were stable. He had omitted only her temperature, so Maureen touched Emily's skin to sense it herself. Normal. The trauma bay had all the equipment needed for a "crash intubation" or "surgical airway." Now she needed the personnel to perform these potential interventions.

The emergency doctor came into the trauma bay.

"Maureen, what do we got?"

He knew whom to ask.

Maureen's reply was short and to the point. Dr. Michael Belleville would only have a brief interaction with Emily. He spoke with the patient calmly and listened to her back with a stethoscope to assess the degree of air entry into her lungs. She had stridor, not wheezing. Stridor is difficulty getting air into the lungs, often from a swollen airway. Wheezing is difficulty getting air out of the lungs, often from an asthmatic attack. He thought this was probably an allergic reaction.

Belleville ordered 50 mg of Benadryl and 100 mg of hydrocortisone to be given intravenously. Maureen had already drawn up those medications; she began to inject the liquid drugs into Emily's IV. She emptied the first syringe and, without taking it out of the one-way valve, sucked back a full syringe of the IV fluid and injected that as well, pushing the medications down the line towards the back of her hand and into her blood stream. She gave the next syringe of medications with another "push." Belleville then announced to everyone, "She is stable. I'm calling anaesthesia to evaluate her airway. Call me if she crashes." After less than three minutes with Emily, he left to finish stitching a nine-year-old boy who had gashed his knuckle drying the inside of a glass while doing the dishes with his father.

Emily had not heard the doctor because of the noise of her own breathing. She made a high-pitched "heee" as she tried to suck in air, and then coughed most of it out. The coughing left her completely exhaled, as if someone had hit her in the solar plexus. The desire to draw in a huge breath was overwhelming, but her constricted throat would not allow it. Her tongue felt fat and the muscles in her throat were squeezing, as if someone was strangling her. The coughing was so fierce she had soaked herself in urine, but her breathing was so difficult she had not noticed.

LEO

Leonard Strait had never been more than a two days' drive from where he was born. Standing six feet, two inches and weighing nearly three hundred pounds, he lived on a small farm in northern British Columbia, near a town called Bear Lake. It was an hour from the nearest regional hospital in Prince George. Leo had made the 150-kilometre round trip many times.

In 2010, Leo had begun to have choking episodes for no reason. Country-raised, he opted for good, old-fashioned stoicism. He dismissed the initial symptoms even when these annoying muscle spasms occurred once every other month. They would last for a few seconds, so it was close to bearable. But then they began to occur every week and last for a minute. He described feeling the left side of his throat squeeze intermittently.

There was nothing in any medical texts to explain this phenomenon. When his family doctor could not recognize or identify these symptoms, Leo was referred to an ears, nose and throat (ENT) specialist.

Intermittent throat contractions are not an uncommon problem for an ENT specialist. Their patients frequently complain of involuntary throat contractions because any irritant in the larynx can cause such a reaction, often called laryngospasm. The most common irritant is an airborne pollutant, for instance, the smoky air following a forest fire or the far more intense difficulty of trying to breathe following exposure to bear spray.

When Leo went to see his first ENT specialist in Prince George, the office had a dozen chairs in the waiting room, all filled, mostly by mothers with their children. Leo felt he didn't belong. He was too big, too old, and he was alone. He filled out the health questionnaire with its long list of medical conditions. "Do you have allergies?" "Do you have asthma?" Leo left them blank. These were boxes that would be ticked by most pediatric clientele. He scanned down the page and began to tick the lower, rarely marked boxes. "Do you have high blood pressure?" "Do you have diabetes?" "Do you have acid reflux?" Yes, yes, yes.

When it was his turn, Leo was ushered into room number 2 to wait for the doctor. The consultant came through the door, reading Leo's referral letter from his family doctor and the attached records from his latest emergency room visit. Leo began to describe his choking and coughing episodes. Their eyes did not meet.

The doctor looked in Leo's throat, ears, and finally up his nose with a light attached to different disposable specula. He determined that Leo's problem had no perceivable link to any common irritant.

The doctor spoke as he wrote a prescription.

"You have acid reflux causing your choking. This is a prescription for a strong antacid. Take one pill twice a day for a month and come back and see me. You can make an appointment on your way out."

After a ten-minute consultation, the doctor was out the door. Leo left the office with the correct prescription for the wrong problem.

At the end of that day, the ENT specialist had seen sixty-four patients: twenty-seven with ear infections, twenty-four with allergies, twelve with sinusitis—and one with a condition that would not be described for another two years.

EMILY

Arthur backed away from the stretcher and sank into a chair facing Emily. He had heard the doctor and did not think Emily was "stable." The casual addition of "call me if she crashes" suggested it was quite possible. He had seen these attacks before over the last five years, but none had been this intense. This scenario was over his head. Arthur began to feel terrible about being momentarily pleased by the severity of this episode, ashamed he was not being more emotionally supportive.

He sat very still and tried to be invisible.

There was a flurry of activity around Emily. Within a few minutes she had a second IV in her arm and an oxygen mask over her mouth. To Arthur it looked as if steam was pouring out; it was humidified air with a higher than normal concentration of oxygen. Meanwhile wires attached to small, circular pads stuck on Emily's chest and shoulders led to an electrocardiograph that beeped out her heart rhythm. Blood was being drawn from her other arm. A second nurse had begun charting the results.

Emily was oblivious to all this activity. She just sucked hard to get air; it was like trying to breathe through a shrinking straw. She later told me the sensation of smothering to death was horrific. Emily's eyes looked wild in response to the adrenalin now circulating through her body, a look Maureen knew. It was panic and it would not last much longer. Patients inevitably tire.

Dressed in green surgical scrubs, the anaesthesiologist stepped into the trauma bay. Dr. Brent Powers was six feet, four inches, fit and imposing. At age sixty, his close-cropped grey hair and youngish face gave little indication of the extraordinary life he had lived. He had trained in South Africa but left during the diaspora under Apartheid. Nothing in Canada had ever come close to the carnage he had seen at Baragwanath Hospital in Soweto. He had removed a half-buried machete from the skull of a screaming child. He had seen death from both violence and neglect. Despite these experiences, or perhaps in response to them, he projected a charming, gregarious demeanour.

There were now six people around Emily, including Dr. Powers, who spoke slowly in a manner that belied the urgency of the situation.

"Well, well, hello. Maureen, what do you have for me?"

"Did you get any info from Michael?"

"Just that there was an airway in one," replied Powers in his Afrikaans accent. He snapped the wrists of his blue latex gloves as he put them on.

"That's it?" Maureen asked, with more than a touch of incredulity and an upward flick of her eyes.

"Is there more?" Powers was a master at reading people. He knew Maureen was very good and he would trust whatever she said.

Both paramedics had moved out once Powers announced himself. That left Maureen on Emily's left side, the second nurse on her right, a respiratory therapist at the head of the bed and Dr. Powers at the foot. He could see from the monitors that Emily was struggling and would not last another five minutes. Her heart rate was 145 beats per minute. This abnormally fast rate (called tachycardia) was a response to adrenalin produced by the stress of her situation. Her respiratory rate was at least 30 per minute, but each breath was very shallow. She was "satting" 100 percent on almost pure oxygen.

"Has she had any Benadryl or steroids?" he asked.

"Given." Maureen replied.

"Ventolin?"

"In the humidifier," the respiratory therapist replied.

Ventolin was used to open airways during asthmatic attacks. Emily did not have asthma, but the medication would not hurt her.

"Open the crash cart," Powers said. He looked at the respiratory therapist. "What IV do we have?"

"Two. A 16 antecubital and an 18 in her hand," Maureen replied before the therapist could answer.

"I'll need a number 7 tube."

Powers moved to Emily's right and pulled her right hand away from her neck. He looked at her name bracelet and felt for her pulse.

"Emily"—he spoke her name as if he was meeting an old friend at a reunion—"are you getting tired?"

Emily nodded but could not speak.

"I'm going to put a small tube in your throat so you can relax and breathe easily." He spoke so matter-of-factly that Emily believed him. But the procedure would require him to paralyze her and, during that moment when she was paralyzed, push an endotracheal tube down her throat between her vocal cords. Once she was paralyzed, she would be unable to breathe by herself. If he could not insert the tube, she would be dead within a few minutes.

"We will give you a little relaxation medication and then slide the tube in. Easy-peasy, lemon-squeezy."

Powers put one hand on Emily's chest and another behind her neck, and pushed her from sitting to lying flat. Emily reached for the sidebars and then to her throat. Powers moved her right arm back down to her side. She reached up again, and he pushed her arm back down. She understood and clenched her fists. He moved around to the head of the stretcher and was now towering over her head.

The ventilator, a machine that could breathe for a patient, was used in every operating room. One was always kept in the emergency room for just such an occasion. Between the mechanical bellows and the plastic tubes leading to the patient was a rubber bag constantly filled with air that could be squeezed by hand to force air into the patient. Powers held the mask over Emily's face with his right hand and "bagged" her with his left. Squeezing the bag to move the air, he could feel how hard it was to push air into her lungs. Air was escaping between the mask and her face. He pushed the mask harder onto her face with his palm and reached under the angle of her jaw to squeeze the mask tighter.

"Let's just bag her for a minute." He spoke through clenched teeth because of the effort, although his tone was still relaxed. "When was the last time she ate?" No one answered—no one was sure whom he was asking. Maureen called over to Arthur, who had remained sitting beside them, out of the way.

"Hey, husband!" She had forgotten his name. "When did she last eat?"

"Ah . . . suppertime. She ate at six." Powers knew Emily's stomach would still be full of food. This was a danger because once he paralyzed her, the liquid contents of her stomach could reflux back up into her throat and then down into her lungs. Aspiration. The acid of the stomach would then begin to digest her lungs.

Powers stopped bagging Emily and injected 10 cc of propofol into her IV. A white liquid with a very rapid anaesthetic effect, propofol is infamous as the drug that killed Michael Jackson.

"You're going to fall asleep now," Powers said, as he injected the drug. Emily was unconscious in a few seconds. He did not bag her anymore for fear of pushing air into her stomach and inducing an aspiration; instead he let her coast. For a brief period, her oxygen saturation would remain normal, because breathing pure oxygen for several minutes had supersaturated her blood and hemoglobin with the

life-sustaining gas. Like a free diver, she could last three or four minutes before the oxygen saturation monitor would alarm.

As she lay on her back, Powers inserted a laryngoscope into her
mouth and pulled up, lifting her tongue upwards against her lower
teeth. Her whole head lifted slightly off the stretcher, and he could see
below the blade down her illuminated throat. Her vocal cords were
surprisingly easy to see. Two vertical pink lips gapping open, not
unlike the labia majora.

Maureen passed him the endotracheal tube. Never taking his eyes
away from the cords, he slipped the clear plastic endotracheal tube down
her throat, past her cords into her trachea. Easy-peasy, lemon-squeezy.

The tubes leading to the face mask were quickly disconnected and
attached to the endotracheal tube. Powers flipped the switch on the ventilator and it began to breathe for her. He scanned the monitors and they
were all normal. No hint of pathology. Sats—normal; airway pressure—
normal. Her throat had looked normal. No swollen tongue, no signs of
allergy. Nothing. The tension in the trauma bay dissipated in an instant.

Powers laughed, "Well, that was a lot easier than I thought." He
looked up and raised both hands like a calf roper at a rodeo signalling
he was done. Then he wrapped a shoelace-like cotton tie around
Emily's neck and tied the endotracheal tube in place before double-
checking the respirator's breaths were appropriate for someone Emily's
size. He pulled the blue latex glove off his left hand and, still holding
it with his right, stretched the cuff of his right glove off his hand,
inverting the glove around the balled-up left one. Pointing the
stretched glove with his thumb at the garbage bin against the far wall,
he let go and fired the gloves. They arced across the room, hit the wall
above the garbage and dropped in.

"And another two points for the conversion," he said. Dr. Powers was
mildly euphoric, enjoying the release of tension. He left the trauma bay to

find Dr. Belleville. Emily lay flaccid on the stretcher, only her chest and abdomen moving up as the bellows emptied rhythmically with a hiss.

LEO

Leo was not the sort of patient prone to undertaking hours of research on the internet, hoping to find answers that had escaped medical staff. But over time he would become familiar with his basic physiology.

The back of the throat, or pharynx, divides into two tubes or passageways: one to the lungs and one to the stomach. The one leading to the lungs, called the larynx, contains the voice box. It continues deeper into the chest as the trachea, which is a ridged tube just under the skin below the Adam's apple, then splits into the two lungs. The other passageway from the throat is the esophagus, a muscular tube leading to the stomach.

The voice box contains the vocal cords. Coordinated contractions of the muscles connected to them change their tension, allowing the cords to vibrate at different frequencies and providing the fundamental sound properties for speech. The larynx's other job is to protect the lungs. Irritants in the larynx can trigger a closure of the vocal cords to stop anything getting into the lungs below. The muscles that activate this closure are the fastest in the body. The larynx can therefore produce both the most sophisticated movement of the human body, a soprano's solo, and its simplest, closure of the throat.

Leo would also learn there are three common causes of episodic throat contractions: inhaled irritants, acid reflux, and the physical manifestation of an underlying psychiatric problem. The last of these is both the most interesting and the least understood.

Leo had been diagnosed with acid reflux causing episodic laryngospasm. The concept is quite simple: acid from the stomach occasionally refluxes back up the esophagus, which can cause a burning sensation deep to the sternum, known as heartburn. If the acid gets further up and into the throat, it can irritate the larynx. The larynx then does its job and closes; the result is called laryngospasm.

Exposure to stomach acid, outside the stomach, is a dangerous thing. It's amazing that the stomach does not eat itself, but its lining is designed to withstand the acidic onslaught. The esophagus, on the other hand, is not. After chronic exposure to acid, its cellular composition changes and predisposes the patient to esophageal cancer.

Bulimia has a similar consequence: the frequent vomiting of stomach acid creates a predisposition to esophageal cancer. How laryngopharyngeal reflux causes laryngospasm is not clear, it just does—presumably by causing an inflammation in the tissues of the larynx. What is clear, however, is that blocking stomach acid can fix the problem.

With his prescription to treat acid reflux, Leo's occasional heartburn stopped. But his choking continued. Leo returned to the ENT specialist several times. Each time the visit was slightly shorter, and it always ended in another prescription for omeprazole (a powerful acid blocker).

As his symptoms continued to worsen, two new problems arose. First, the episodes were starting to occur while he was sleeping. Second, some of them were severe enough that he could not catch his breath.

During a typical choking episode, the muscles on the left side of his throat would squeeze rock-hard. His wife, Sophia, had felt the muscles during such a spasm and knew the symptoms were consistently left-sided.

It was around this time, however, that Leo noticed that some of the spasms were circumferential—that is, it was as if someone was squeezing both sides of his neck with their hands. One of these episodes sent Leo to the emergency, thinking he might die of suffocation. When he arrived by ambulance, the charge nurse called a code blue, and Leo was rushed into the resuscitation bay and quickly surrounded by a team of healthcare workers.

The doctor looked at Leo and then at the charge nurse. Leo now looked fine and the nurse looked uncomfortable. His spasms had spontaneously stopped, just as they always had in the past, and he was sitting up, breathing quietly, and satting 100 percent with an oxygen mask.

The doctor pulled the mask off Leo's face with a roughness that more than hinted at his displeasure for this false alarm. The team left the room one at a time, and Leo was left with a young nurse who charted his vitals and listened to his story. Several hours later, the emergency physician returned.

"I've been reading your chart," he began. "And these episodes have been going on for some time."

"Yes."

Leo was by nature a straightforward man, the definition of taciturn.

"Have you got a lot of stress in your life?" the doctor asked, clearly exploring the diagnosis of a psychiatric disorder.

"This choking is stressful."

"I mean before the choking started. Did you have a trauma in your life?"

"No."

The doctor did not have the time to explore Leo's psyche. He wrote a referral for a psychiatric consultation, and it was left to the young nurse to explain to Leo and Sophia that these symptoms might be coming from psychological stress. Leo could not think what that might be. He obligingly said, "Okay."

When he and Sophia were driving home, Leo had to pull over for another spasm. This one was a "one-sider," the kind that squeezed the left side of his neck. The squeezing never hurt, but it came with coughing that was severe enough that he had to stop driving. Leo had not spoken much about the coughing because the doctors were always more interested in the choking. Almost every time there was choking, he'd experience a tickling sensation deep to the notch in the front of his neck, which would trigger a cough that often made him see stars. When the coughing was particularly severe, he would get a bad headache afterwards.

Leo and Sophia drove home once the coughing stopped.

The next week he was back in an ambulance. This time the choking had started while he was sleeping and was more than just a one-sider. He could feel his windpipe getting smaller. By the time they reached the emergency department, he was really struggling to breathe. He clutched desperately at his throat. This was the worst he had ever felt, and it was terrifying.

But like the boy who cried wolf, Leo had unwittingly outstayed his welcome at that emergency department. Despite his natural stoicism and clear descriptions of his problem, the last note in his chart read "psychological problem." Leo was patronizingly soothed by the admitting nurse, who told him, "It will get better soon." She began to ask a series of questions: "Do you have any allergies?" "Are you on any medications?" "Do you have any medical problems?" "Is your wife with you?"

But Leo could not answer. He could not breathe; he felt his throat completely close and coughed out his last breath. The room darkened and he fainted back onto the gurney.

EMILY

Drs. Powers and Belleville had a brief conversation that would set back Emily's diagnosis for another year. After reviewing her dramatic symptoms and lack of physical findings, they concluded her problem was likely psychosomatic.

Belleville allowed the paralyzing agents to wear off and removed Emily's endotracheal tube within the hour. She was a different woman. Calm, breathing normally and apologetic. The miraculous transformation confirmed Belleville's opinion that the problem had been psychosomatic to begin with.

Before she left, Belleville spoke to Emily. "Your symptoms don't fit with any breathing problem related to your lungs or throat. They are likely coming from a neurological problem." He took care to avoid the phrase "it's all in your head." He wanted Emily and Arthur to accept the diagnosis and not balk at the psychiatric cause.

"A neurological problem?" Arthur echoed.

"Yes."

"What kind of problem?" Emily asked, her voice hoarse from the evening's trauma.

"That will need an expert to sort out. I am referring you to one of our psychiatrists, Dr. Chip Esparto."

"A psychiatrist?" Arthur wondered why it was not a neurologist.

"Yes. This could be a problem in your subconscious causing these unwanted muscle spasms. There are no signs it's anything else. It's important to rule out everything. Dr. Esparto is an expert in this area."

As he finished talking, Belleville was already reading the details of the next chart. He handed Emily a piece of paper with the psychiatrist's phone number and address, backed out of the emergency bay and pulled the yellow curtains closed behind him.

Emily was physically exhausted and emotionally drained. She wanted to leave. Now on their own, she and Arthur did not speak. Emily straightened her clothes, and together they walked out of the emergency room.

They were standing in the dark parking lot in front of the hospital before Arthur remembered they had arrived by ambulance and ran back inside to order a taxi. Emily, now both literally and figuratively alone, realized her pants were soaking wet and began to cry.

Arthur returned quickly and held her under her arm as if she needed support. She did not. She needed a diagnosis. She knew her choking was real and that it was a physical and not a psychological problem. This last episode had been the worst, and the doctors had told her nothing—again. Apart from a name bracelet around her wrist, the only thing she had got was the small piece of paper with the psychiatrist's name.

She crushed the paper and threw it away.

The couple left in a taxi and returned home with no answers.

———

When Emily got home, she searched "causes of choking" and got a list of 124. The top three causes were "acute mountain sickness," "asthma of pregnancy," and "adult panic-anxiety syndrome." No to all three.

In the days that followed, Emily became an internet student of choking, searching Google, Reddit, Wikipedia, YouTube and even Bing. She read about "vocal cord dysfunction" and "paradoxical vocal fold motion." Adapting her searches to information provided by well-recognized medical institutions, she bookmarked Harvard Medical School and the American Laryngological Association.

Emily was homing in on her problem. The description of vocal cord dysfunction, or VCD, sounded like a good summary of her issues. She shared many of the symptoms: episodic choking, difficulty breathing in, coughing and changes in voice.

People with VCD complain of "difficulty breathing in" or "fighting for breath," they may report a tightness in the throat or chest, and the episodes of shortness of breath are recurrent and can be severe enough to cause unconsciousness. Emily had all three symptoms.

Agitation and a sense of panic were not uncommon and could lead to hospitalization. *Bingo*, she thought.

The more she read about VCD, the more she was convinced she had it. But the treatments for it were all over the place and seemed a bit random. Antacids, steroids, psychotherapy, antidepressants, speech therapy and Botox injections. *Botox injections*?! Emily read that speech therapy reduced 90 percent of emergency room visits by patients with VCD and wondered if that study had been written by a speech therapist hungry for referrals. At the same time, she wondered how to meet a speech therapist. A quick Google search found ten of them nearby. Emily chose the closest one, referred herself and made an appointment for later that week.

That meeting would be the first in a series of events that led her to the cure of her unknown condition.

Dr. Linda Rammage was a speech pathologist based at Vancouver General Hospital at the time. The co-founder of the provincial Voice Care Resource Program, she had specialized in voice science and voice disorders for more than thirty years. Emily had come to the right person—probably the best speech therapist in the country.

Dr. Rammage listened carefully to Emily's story. When Emily finished, she asked additional questions. She excluded a long list of possible aggravating factors and distilled the remaining ones into a shortlist: loud or prolonged talking could trigger a spasm. The odour of harsh chemicals, especially latex, could trigger a spasm. Emily had seen an allergist who had told her she was allergic to latex. Later she would learn that this was not true. The spasms could come spontaneously, and the problem was slowly worsening. She did not have heartburn. She did not have a particularly stressful life, except for the choking.

The questions were surprisingly thorough and uncomfortably intimate. No, she had never been sexually abused. Yes, she was in a loving relationship. Dr. Rammage began to really understand what was common, what was rare, and what never occurred during each of Emily's attacks.

Then Dr. Rammage taught Emily that panting would trick the vocal cords into opening during an attack. The final thing she did was refer Emily to Dr. Murray Morrison, professor of otolaryngology and an international expert in voice disorders.

That was the second event that would lead to her cure.

LEO

Leo awoke to a crowd of people around him. His ears were ringing and he could not yet focus his eyes. There was a tingling heaviness in his limbs and a calm confusion in his head. Leo had passed out because of his choking and coughing. At last, he had convinced the medics that his symptoms were real, but it was a pyrrhic victory: he felt it had nearly cost him his life.

Things changed for Leo from that moment on. He was no longer that "weird guy" with the choking; he was now the guy with the "weird choking." With this reputation, he was referred to an ENT specialist in Vancouver.

The province of British Columbia is nearly four times the size of the United Kingdom but has less than a tenth of its population. Its medical system is built around the primary caregiver—the family doctor—and the government provides financial incentives for young doctors to live in rural communities. They manage what they can and refer what they need help with, typically to a general surgeon or internist in the nearest city. If these specialists encounter problems they are not equipped to manage, the patient then goes to the tertiary care specialist in the nearest major metropolitan area. Many people live a long way from a tertiary care specialist, but there is a travel program that pays for them to get to one if needed.

That is how Leo and Sophia made the trip down to Vancouver and met Dr. Teresa Thermo. With family roots in Italy, she had done most of her training in the United Kingdom, specializing in surgery for head and neck tumours. Dignified and attentive, Thermo greeted the Straits and listened to Leo's story. "I have this choking and coughing that comes and goes. When it comes, the left side of my throat balls up real tight, so I can't breathe." Leo made a fist and held it in front of his throat, to help her understand. Dr. Thermo had not heard a story quite like that before.

Her examination of the patient was purposeful, methodical but ultimately unhelpful. She used a thin grey videoscope to look down his throat through his nose. Everything looked normal. A CT scan would later also be reported as normal. A normal CT was unusual in her oncology practice; usually a blessing, in this case it was disappointing.

Dr. Thermo arranged for Leo to have esophageal pH monitoring—a small tube, placed through his nose into the esophagus, measured the acidity over a two-day period. It had a probe that was placed just above the lower esophageal sphincter above the stomach. If Leo's lower esophagus was full of acid, that would mean he had gastroesophageal reflux disease. The tube had a second probe higher up the esophagus to detect if that part was also exposed to stomach acid and could be causing laryngopharyngeal reflux.

Leo wore the tube in his nose and down his throat for two days, and the pH level in his esophagus never dropped below 4. In fact, he did have gastroesophageal reflux disease—it was just being effectively treated by the omeprazole he'd been prescribed. Leo's occasional heartburn had resolved shortly after taking the medication, but acid reflux was never the cause of his choking.

During the time of these sophisticated tests, Leo's appointment with a psychiatrist came up. He described his ordeal to the psychiatrist with a simple narrative that captured both the frustration of not understanding what was wrong and the anxiety of anticipating the next attack. Leo asked the psychiatrist to send his report to Dr. Thermo, because he felt she was leading the investigation. The concluding sentence encapsulated the psychiatrist's thoughts: "In summary, this gentleman's anxiety and depression are a consequence of his unexplained illness, not the cause of it." Leo was prescribed an antidepressant and given a follow-up appointment for one month later. He never filled the prescription and never returned to the psychiatrist. It was a surprising act of defiance for him, but he had had enough.

Dr. Thermo called the Straits into her office and summarized her diagnostic findings: there was nothing wrong except for his life-threatening choking episodes. The good news was there was no tumour, no acid reflux, no asthma, no allergies, no neurological illness and no psychiatric cause.

The bad news was that Dr. Thermo could offer Leo only one option—a tracheostomy, a recommendation that alarmed him. Years before, he had seen an anti-smoking advertisement on TV. There was a withered, elderly lady in a wheelchair, clearly near death, still smoking by putting her cigarette into the open hole of her tracheostomy in her throat. Her seemingly resigned indifference to death and the continuance of her addiction despite her disfigurement had shaken Leo. He had stopped smoking that very day. Now Dr. Thermo was suggesting he, too, should have a permanent plastic tube go through a small hole in his lower throat, linking the outside air directly to his trachea and bypassing his throat, larynx and vocal cords. Leo was scared by both the disfiguring surgery and the realization that he had no choice but to accept it.

Dr. Thermo explained the benefits and risks of the procedure, which she had performed hundreds of times. Leo wondered if, like the elderly smoker, he was destined to die from his condition.

Two weeks later, Leonard Strait had his tracheostomy. After the successful procedure, Dr. Thermo met him in the recovery room and spoke to him while he lay on the stretcher. "The operation went fine," she said. "Now you have a plastic tube through your throat with a cork on the outside. When you get a choking episode, you can open the cork on your trach to breathe. When it's over, put the cork back in so you can speak." Leo thought she sounded disappointed.

Dr. Thermo had always been the brightest child, the top student, the best surgeon. She was comfortable with excellence. But this case was humbling. She had spent her career saving and losing patients with terrible cancers. She had spoken with many families about a horrendous prognosis or the need for disfiguring facial surgery. And yet this case struck her as unusually discomforting. Technically it had been a successful operation and she had helped the patient to the best of her ability, but she was utterly unsatisfied—a feeling reflected in her parting words to him: "I still don't really know what's wrong with you."

EMILY

Professor Murray Morrison was a very tall man with white hair and a youthful grin. He was always smiling and infused with optimism, projecting the confidence of a man who had been very good at what he did for a very long time. Now a few months away from retirement, he had built a career as a laryngologist treating primarily disorders of the voice. An accomplished singer himself and a member of the Vancouver Bach Choir for many years, he saw all the professional singers in British Columbia who needed medical care. Although he was too modest to ever mention it, it was rumoured Katharine Hepburn had seen him when she'd developed throat cancer. He was that good.

Dr. Rammage felt Emily could have VCD, and Dr. Morrison was seeing her to make sure there was nothing more serious, like laryngeal cancer. His examination revealed no abnormalities. He sprayed the back of her throat with a local anaesthetic and then put a thin laryngoscope into her mouth and peered down her windpipe. Morrison held her tongue and directed the scope with his other hand. Seated on her right side, he looked up and over her right shoulder at a flat-screen monitor behind her that showed a high-definition video of what the laryngoscope could see. He asked Emily to say "eee" and watched her vocal cords move. She gagged a few times, but Morrison saw what he wanted and removed the scope. Nothing out of the ordinary.

When Dr. Rammage next saw Emily, she directed her to begin a program of breathing exercises and to come see her every week. After a month, Emily desperately wanted to tell her she was better, but she was not. Her choking continued. She was choking at least once or twice a week, and sometimes it would awaken her. Her dreams always revolved around drowning just before the closure of her throat would wake her up.

Dr. Rammage referred her back to Morrison for consideration of Botox injections. Botox was more famous for its anti-wrinkle effect, but it had a number of less superficial uses. The active ingredient is Botulinum toxin, the same bacterial poison responsible for botulism, a lethal food poisoning still occasionally seen following ingestion of improperly canned foods. The toxin is the most powerful poison known. Two nanograms per kilogram can kill the average person (a single gram, too small to see, could theoretically kill a million people). That had not been lost on the wayward scientists working for the Nazis, Imperial Japan, and today's who's who of biological weaponizers. It is more powerful than ricin, anthrax, sarin and tetrodotoxin. The discovery of Botulinum toxin in the early 1800s was the first clear description of a food-borne illness—a revolutionary concept back then. Only half a century earlier, witches had been blamed for the symptoms that followed botulism.

For more than twenty years, Dr. Morrison had used Botox to temporarily paralyze one of the vocal cords and weaken the muscle contractions associated with VCD. After he injected the right vocal cord of Emily's throat, her voice was hoarse for a few weeks. Without the full movement of her right vocal cord, air was able to escape from between her vocal cords when she talked, causing a breathy voice. Once her voice recovered, the still-weakened right side of her throat could not contract as hard during a choking episode. Her choking still occurred, but at one-tenth of the intensity. At first she waited for the symptoms to return, but they did not. Emily could not believe it was finally over. Eventually she began to trust that the treatment had worked, and for the first time in a year, she went to bed without fear. Finally she slept without waking to a drowning sensation.

Two months later, the severity of Emily's choking episodes began to increase again, and she went back to see Dr. Morrison. Morrison repeated the Botox injection. He would continue to inject Emily's right throat every two months for the next year. It worked every time. She would have a few weeks of a breathy voice and then a month with very little choking. But then the symptoms would gradually escalate, prompting the next injection, which was effective but uncomfortable and occasionally painful. Ultimately this was a band-aid solution, temporarily covering up the symptoms but not curing the problem.

The Canadian medical system has strengths and weaknesses. The strength is you will receive care regardless of your ability to pay. If Bryan Cranston's character from *Breaking Bad*, Walter White, lived in Canada, he would get his chemotherapy for free and the impetus for his criminal career—medical bankruptcy—would never have existed. The weakness of the system is you will have to wait for that care. Eight months after her first appointment with Dr. Morrison, the radiology department called Emily to schedule the MRI he had ordered. It is common to wait eight months to a year for an MRI.

Emily's MRI revealed an unusually large blood vessel on the right side of her brainstem. Dr. Morrison needed to talk to a brain expert about the possible significance of that vessel. Could it be the cause of her problems?

This was the third consultation that would lead her to a cure.

6.

THE DISCOVERY OF HELPS

I first met Emily on October 21, 2014. As I listened to her story, my concern for her was overwhelmed by a growing excitement I tried to contain.

When I began my neurosurgical practice in 1995, I was familiar with the neurovascular compression syndromes—the result of a blood vessel pounding against a cranial nerve—and how to cure them with an operation called microvascular decompression, or MVD. Compression of the fifth cranial nerve (the sensory nerve to the face) causes trigeminal neuralgia, or intermittent facial pain. Compression of the seventh cranial nerve (the motor nerve to the face) causes intermittent facial spasms. Compression of the ninth cranial nerve (the sensory nerve to the throat) causes glossopharyngeal neuralgia, or intermittent throat pain. MVD was designed to decompress the affected nerve and relieve the symptoms. I had wondered for years if the compression of the tenth cranial nerve (the motor nerve to the throat) could cause intermittent spasms of the throat, but none of my colleagues had ever heard of such a thing. It was a missing syndrome in my mind; it should exist. As I continued to listen to Emily, I wondered if she could be the patient I had been waiting to meet for the last twenty years.

Dr. Morrison had referred Emily to me because my area of interest was stereotactic and functional neurosurgery, a subspeciality that includes all the neurovascular compression syndromes. It was Felix Durity's idea for us to subspecialize in Vancouver. In his generation, everybody did everything—but he knew that focusing on a few problems would generate experts in those areas. My knowledge and curiosity about this facet of neurosurgery were a direct product of Dr. Durity's vision.

Functional neurosurgery also specializes in the surgical treatment of Parkinson's disease, which has undergone revolutionary advancements in recent decades. Since the 1950s, neurosurgeons had been destroying the parts of the brain causing Parkinsonian tremors or stiffness. In the 1990s, the new technology of deep brain stimulation allowed us to modulate the activity of these brain areas with electricity instead of destroying the tissue, which dramatically reduced the complications associated with the surgical treatment of Parkinson's disease. When we used to destroy the brain regions with heat, there was no way to reverse a complication. If the lesion was slightly too big, patients suffered the resultant complication for the rest of their life. With DBS, the effect could be adjusted to fit the individual patient's need. Turn up the stimulation if the effects are too weak, turn down the stimulation if there is a side effect. I had started our deep brain stimulation program in 1999.

Recently, I received a thank-you email from a patient whose arm tremor, from a condition called essential tremor, had stopped when I turned on their deep brain stimulator. During his brain surgery, there was a moment when I tested the stimulator to make sure it could block the tremor without any side effects. The patient was awake during this operation (tremor stops when you are asleep), and I held up my finger and asked him to touch it. With the DBS turned on, he reached up and touch my fingertip with a steady hand.

"Now stay there," I asked, and he did. It was the first time his tremor had ceased in forty years. After thirty seconds or so, I said, "Now I'm going to turn off the stimulator." Within a few moments, his hand shook wildly away from my steady fingertip. Just then he burst into tears. The moment was overwhelming for him. I reassured him that many patients get emotional at that instant when they realize what the technology can do when it is placed perfectly in their brain. His email to me had a picture of Michelangelo's *Creation of Adam* and he wrote, "This is how I felt last week." The famous painting adorning the ceiling of the Sistine Chapel has God reaching out and touching Adam's fingertip to give him "the spark of life."

This technology has had extraordinary benefits, allowing patients with Parkinson's disease to walk again. As the only surgeon providing that operation in a province of five million people, I now have one of the largest reservoirs of personal experience with DBS in the world. Dr. Durity was right; specialization brought experience and experience brought expertise.

A few years into my practice, my senior colleague, Dr. Ian Turnbull, retired, and I inherited from him a large cohort of patients with trigeminal neuralgia. Far more excruciating than childbirth or kidney stones, TN, as we call it, is frequently described as the most painful condition the human body can experience. Before physicians developed treatments, it had been given the moniker "the suicide disease." The cause is often a blood vessel near the brainstem pinching or pressing on the trigeminal nerve, which normally conveys pain and touch sensation from one side of your face to your brain. It has many tiny branches, which innervate your teeth as well as all the skin of the face. With the recognition that TN could be caused by a blood vessel pinching the trigeminal nerve came the realization that it could be cured by moving that vessel away and decompressing the nerve. In 1995 I began to practise MVD to relieve TN.

MVD is a beautiful operation. To look down the microscope during MVD is to see one of God's greatest creations. The anatomy of the brainstem is packed with unique structures and is as visually stunning as it is complex. Because the problem being addressed is a blood vessel—not the distorted anatomy of trauma or a tumour—the surgeon's view is pristine. The goal of surgery is to move the vessel off the nerve and thereby decompress the nerve.

After performing several hundred MVD operations, mostly for compression of the fifth cranial nerve causing TN, I began to wonder what would happen if a blood vessel compressed the tenth cranial nerve—the vagus nerve. Compression of the sixth cranial nerve to the eye muscles, causing double vision, was incredibly rare—I had operated on only one patient with it. Compression of the seventh nerve to the muscles of the face causes hemifacial spasm and was a common surgery for me. Compression of the eighth cranial nerve to the ear could cause tinnitus but was very rare and difficult to diagnose (many things cause tinnitus). Compression of the ninth nerve to the throat causes glosso-pharyngeal neuralgia and is also very rare, but I had done more than a dozen of these operations. Compression of the tenth cranial nerve, the vagus nerve, causes . . . well, I had never heard anyone talk about it. The vagus nerve includes fibres to the muscles of the throat, and compres-sion of the vagus nerve *should* cause spasms on one side of the throat. Like hemifacial spasm, only in the throat—hemi-throat spasm.

Dr. Morrison had told me there was a large vessel on the right side of Emily's brainstem, so I wondered if Emily could be describing hemi-throat spasm. Unfortunately her symptoms did not completely fit; she described her choking as being circumferential, not one-sided.

As hard as I tried, I could not get her to agree that her symptoms were lateralized to the right. She was very clear in her description: the choking was like someone wrapping their hands around her neck and squeezing. These intermittent throat spasms were slowly progressing in strength, frequency and duration, but they were not worse on the right, did not start on the right, and did not last longer on the right. She felt they were equal on both sides.

I sank back in my chair. Her symptoms did not exactly fit with what I was looking for. Maybe she was not the one who would validate my theory about the compression of the tenth cranial nerve. But maybe she was. One of her most compelling symptoms, I thought, was the fact that her throat spasms could occur while sleeping. Nothing psychological could cause a spasm while the brain slept. Only a physical problem could do that.

On her MRI there was a large vessel near the right vagus nerve. Morrison's Botox treatments on the right side had almost eliminated her symptoms, so that sounded one-sided. Maybe, I thought, people can only describe throat contractions as being circumferential; maybe patients can't distinguish a left or right throat contraction. If that was the case, it all could fit.

I phoned Morrison as soon as Emily had left and asked him why he chose the right side of her neck for the Botox. He said it was pure habit. The patients sit in his examination chair and he usually sits on a stool in front of them on their right side. He is right-handed and as he leans in close to them, their right neck is the closest side to inject the Botox.

I pulled up Emily's MRI—an anatomical picture of the brain performed in slices—on my desktop. The computer can scroll through these slices sequentially, so you can build up a three-dimensional image of the brain and its blood vessels in your mind. The resolution of the MRI is such that it can see the bigger trigeminal and facial nerves, which are about three millimetres in diameter, quite well. The vagus nerve, however, is made up of five or six much smaller rootlets that join together to form the tenth cranial nerve. These rootlets are about a millimetre in diameter and are often too small to see on the MRI (especially if the patient moves slightly during the procedure).

This was the case with Emily. On one of her MRI sequences, I could see the abnormally large posterior inferior cerebellar artery (one of the three main arteries that supply the cerebellum) on the right side of Emily's brain, but I could not see her vagus nerve. On a different MRI sequence, I could just make out the vagus nerve but not the vessel distorting the nerve.

I copied both the images, one showing the nerve and the other showing the vessel, into a PowerPoint presentation and then ran them as a slide show. Flipping between the two images, I could see that the location of the vessel overlapped exactly with the location of the nerve.

A curving vessel, just like a water hose, always pulses outwards in the direction of blood flow. The convex side of the vessel's curve moves outwards with each heartbeat and, if there is a nerve against it, will rub against it. Over the course of several decades, the insulation (myelin) of that nerve can be damaged or rubbed off, causing the nerve to short-circuit and leading to unwanted signals in the nerve—electrical pain if it is the trigeminal nerve or muscle twitching if it is the facial nerve. There is an ongoing battle between any vessel and the nerve it abuts. The vessel is continually rubbing off the myelin; the nerve is continually trying to heal. Over time the vessel tends to win. The vessel slowly gets firmer due to aging, and the nerve's ability to heal lessens with aging.

All the information was now in front of me. There were no more tests available. It was time to decide.

To operate or not to operate, that was the question.

I reviewed Emily's case again. She suffered from intermittent choking that continued even when she was asleep. This was crucial; it ruled out a psychogenic cause.

The mind is a very powerful instrument that can cause illness when it needs to. Your subconscious, for example, may protect your conscious mind from the memory of a previous horror. The Holocaust survivor who loses their sense of smell may be saved from an odour that reminds them of the atrocities. The abused child who becomes paralyzed can no longer be asked to fetch the belt used to beat them.

Psychoanalysts have studied psychogenic illnesses and understand how powerful and debilitating the effects of the mind can be on the body. Patients are completely unaware their disabilities are caused by their unconscious mind and not a physical illness. They are not faking their condition—that would be called malingering. Sigmund Freud coined the term "conversion disorder" for this psychogenic condition; he tried to find the root cause of the psychological trauma and, by acknowledging it, end the need for its defensive illness.

Choking can be psychogenic. The primitive reflex of protecting the lungs or stomach from something entering the body is a not uncommon manifestation of conversion disorder. One of the hallmarks of these disorders is that they are distractible. When the patient is asked to focus on a complex mental problem, their "paralyzed" leg may begin to move. Conversion disorders also do not occur while sleeping. The complex mind capable of fooling the body into paralysis or blindness rests every night. Patients with a conversion disorder causing paralysis can sleepwalk, roll over in bed, and freely move their legs into a more comfortable position while asleep.

Only one intermittent muscle-twitching condition that I was aware of could occur while sleeping—and that was hemifacial spasm. This twitching of one side of the face is caused by a blood vessel pinching the seventh cranial nerve near the brainstem, and it can be cured by MVD surgery and decompression of the nerve. If there was a hemi-throat spasm condition caused by compression of the tenth cranial nerve—the vagus nerve—it should also occur while sleeping. The analogy between Emily's choking and hemifacial spasm began to deepen in my mind.

Hemifacial spasm can be treated with Botox injections into the affected facial muscles, and Emily's choking was dramatically improved with Botox injections on the right side of her throat. Hemifacial spasm always has a vessel that can be seen on an MRI pressing on the facial nerve. Flipping back and forth in the PowerPoint presentation had shown that Emily had a vessel right where her vagus nerve should be.

Therefore her condition *should* be cured if I moved that vessel away. Everything fit except her description of her choking. It should have been one-sided, not circumferential. I tried outlining my thoughts to her. "I think I know why you are choking, and I think I can cure it." But my explanation was long-winded and defensive. I think she must have stopped listening after I said, "I think I can cure it."

Emily signed the consent form and was booked for surgery in three months' time.

7.

THE OPERATION

mily entered Vancouver General at 5:30 a.m. on January 30, 2015. Her husband had driven her. It was still dark out at that hour, and Vancouver's winter rain was continuously drizzling. The couple had not talked much—no pep talk or advice. Just, "I'll park and meet you at admitting."

The admitting clerk wrapped a blue identification bracelet around Emily's right wrist and gave her directions to the surgical pre-admission care centre. Emily waited in the hallway for Arthur, then they took the elevator up to the second floor.

The hospital was still quiet and the hallway surprisingly dim and deserted. Following the signs, they pushed through a door into a large, very bright room with multiple curtained-off stretchers around the perimeter and desks with computers in the middle. The scene was frenetic, with all the nurses in green scrubs doing something in haste. The patients were lying on stretchers wearing gowns and looking lost, stoic or scared.

Emily introduced herself to the nurse standing just inside the entrance. She reached for Emily's wristband, read the name, checked her clipboard and pointed to an empty stretcher across the room. "You're in Bay 12," was all she said. Emily and Arthur walked over there without talking.

At Bay 12 Emily was immediately greeted by another nurse, who pulled her behind the curtains and closed them. She helped Emily change into a gown and asked her a series of questions. "When was the last time you ate?" "Do you have any allergies?" "Are you taking any medications?"

Emily had answered most of these questions several days before when she'd met an anaesthesiologist in the pre-admission clinic. Engineers had developed the safety of redundancy to reduce the chance of failure in a given system. The airline industry had perfected this system long ago with back-up systems and double-checks; medicine was only recently following aviation's lead. Within fifteen minutes, Emily was gowned and ready. She had an IV inserted into the back of her left hand, and the curtains were pulled back.

I met her at 7 a.m. She was reclining on the stretcher, with the covers pulled up to her neck. Arthur sat in a chair by her side. We greeted each other, and I set out to put them at ease. We had already reviewed and agreed upon the risks and rewards long ago; now it was time to optimize the surgery.

"My anaesthesiologist will meet you and ask a bunch of questions you've already answered, and then we'll take you into the room. It's about a three-hour operation, but they don't rush me. We'll take our time, and you'll be fast asleep the whole time."

"Okay."

"I understand that it is a big day for you guys, but it's just another Friday for me." They nodded. "Any questions?"

"No. We're good," Arthur replied.

"I need to sign you on the right, so everyone knows what side we're operating on." I tore a purple marker out of its sterile plastic cover and wrote "CH" on her right shoulder. "You'll be asked a bunch of times what side the surgery is, so don't be surprised or worried as if we don't know."

I reached for her hand. "We'll take good care of you." And I left to prepare the operating room.

I am a slow surgeon. I prefer cutting what I can see, then pausing to retract the brain so I can see better. I think this approach could have stemmed from a fear of failure—or put another way, I absolutely hate to lose. Competing in athletics, I had taken little pleasure in winning but hated coming second. When I ran track, my fastest times were in lane 8. Lane 8 is the furthest outside; the runner starts staggered slightly ahead, since the inside lanes have a shorter distance around the corners. Starting a bit in front, you cannot see your competitors. You run scared until the last bend, when the distances are evened out and the runners are side by side. When I was in lane 1, with everyone ahead of me at the start, I felt I was running angry and the outcome was never as strong. Fear of losing made me run faster.

My cautious approach to surgery was also likely affected by participating in competitive diving in university and eventually at the Olympics. I was always thinking about what could go wrong with the dive instead of relaxing and letting it just happen. The cerebral cortex, where thinking is performed, is too slow to correctly affect the outcome of a complex dive. The control of the muscles must come from the cerebellum, the "little brain" that sits at the back of the head below the cerebrum. The cerebellum works very fast to coordinate muscle activity. Functioning at a subconscious level, it probably reflects what some people call muscle memory.

At some point during my surgical training, the fear of losing had morphed into the fear of something going wrong. At every point in an operation, my recurring thought was, What could go wrong now? If I pulled on a piece of tumour attached to a blood vessel, I thought, When will this vessel break? not When will this piece come off? That fear of a mistake likely reduced my complication rate, but it is a pervasive thought process that cannot be turned off at will.

I worry about everything that is not directly in my control. For instance, flying as a passenger is difficult (unless I'm exhausted or distracted). Driving is easy but oncoming traffic is stressful. Letting our children play outside was challenging. I finished the basement in our first house in Port Moody, but not before mentally rehearsing the response to each unlikely but disfiguring accident with a table saw, nail gun or ripping hammer.

The fear of failure, or of something going wrong, is probably innate and its magnitude set by your genetics. Its effects are widespread and variable. In sports it can either spur you on or inhibit your movements. In surgery it can make you safe or prevent you from trying new difficult manoeuvres. Some say the greatest technical surgeons are all psychopaths—free from the fear of trying something dangerous. These technical wizards can pull that piece of tumour off the blood vessel and dispassionately watch the artery tear and bleed. Their response is, "Now I know how strong those arteries are," not, "Oh my God, the patient is going to be devastated by that stroke." That is not me. I slowly acquired the knowledge of how resilient the brain and its blood vessels were over years of trying just a bit harder. Never over the edge, but creeping asymptotically up to it.

My personality fortunately fit with functional neurosurgery, where the patient is electing to have surgery to improve their quality of life. They are not actively dying of a brain tumour that needs to be removed at all costs (where surgical errors can be justified by the prolonged life). They are not devastated by an injury and in need of surgery to save their life (where surgical errors can be hidden by the initial neurological injury). Patients coming for functional neurosurgery are intact before the operation, and any surgical injury is immediately obvious.

My patients want their facial pain eliminated or their arm tremors reduced, but not at any cost. That was always in the back of my mind when I operated.

I walked into OR number 18. No one was there yet.

I plugged in the microscope and checked its balance. The Zeiss Pentero is a sleek, 1,000-pound, Swiss-made surgical microscope that can magnify images thirty-nine times in stunning clarity. Sometimes looking through the scope at the brain felt like cheating. You could see everything—things I could not see with the naked eye. You could see exactly what to cut and what not to. It would not be hyperbole to say I loved that scope.

The only other pieces of engineering I loved were my Mercedes SUV and my Specialized Enduro mountain bike. The former sounds ostentatious, but every time I was called to emergency to see a seriously injured victim of a motor vehicle accident, I made a point of asking the paramedics what car the patient was driving. During my five years of residency training, there were occasionally luxury cars but never a Mercedes. This small, biased study resulted in the purchase of the SUV a few years before I could afford it. The mountain bike allowed me to ride my favourite, uniquely named trails on the North Shore, Squamish and Whistler. I could not climb "50 Shades of Green" and dared not descend "Pamplemousse," "Business Time," or "Seventh" without it.

The Pentero microscope also enabled photographs and videos to be taken to record what I was seeing and doing. I hoped and believed we would see something important during Emily's surgery. Something that had never been seen before—proof that compression of the tenth nerve causes throat contractions. After setting up the microscope, I began to prepare the positioning equipment.

I had the pleasure of knowing I was doing the work that I was meant to be doing. And I understand that not everyone gets to feel that way. The reasons for my attraction to this profession changed over the years, but I had known I wanted to be a neurosurgeon since grade six. This early fascination became a positive feedback loop that reinforced itself—the more I learned, the more interesting the brain became. In high school, I liked the fact that the brain was the most complex organ; it was not in second place. And following my epiphany in the ER as an intern, the path to neurosurgery became clearer. While doing my doctoral thesis at Oxford, I realized that we know so little about the brain that there was a good chance of discovering something new, and I liked the idea of potentially adding to the knowledge of this remarkable organ. Later still, as a neurosurgical resident, I liked the technical challenge of the operations. I'd felt sure I would easily become bored removing my hundredth appendix, but each neurosurgical operation seemed to have an abundance of unique difficulties.

Finally, as a neurosurgeon, I appreciated neurosurgery because it was a pleasure to work with the people it attracted. Neurosurgery nurses, like those from the emergency department and the intensive care unit, are often the most dedicated, reliable and well trained.

JFK famously said, "We choose to go to the moon in this decade and do the other things, not because they are easy but because they are hard." Kennedy may have been talking about the space race but he was right about life. Some people choose difficult things—such as joining the Marines, climbing Everest or becoming a neurosurgical nurse—because they are hard. Like Betty and Wai-Yee.

Betty would scrub today. She left to wash her hands in the sink outside the OR doors while I talked to Wai-Yee.

"Is the Maquet table okay for this case?" she asked.

"Yes."

"Do you need anything else?"

"I need some more foam for positioning."

That was all I needed to say. I knew for sure she would solve the problem. There was no need to expend additional energy worrying about whether or not she would get what I asked for. That's the joy in working with good colleagues.

The anaesthesiologist, Dr. Elinor Rommany, and her resident entered the room. Rommany specializes in neurosurgery procedures—a neuroanaesthetist. She is superb and a pleasure to work with. Her resident was a large, muscular man in his late twenties with a full beard. He looked more like an orthopaedic surgeon than an anaesthetist. (For years orthopaedic surgeons have relished their blue-collar persona, emphasized by the hammer and saws they use as "instruments" during surgery and their predominantly male demographic—but that is changing, as more women enter the field.)

Elinor and I knew each other very well.

"Do you need anything special for this case?" she asked.

"She is a right MVD," I said, depersonalizing the patient, as is *de rigueur* going into the operation. "I will be working around the vagus and could cause bradycardia."

Bradycardia is the slowing of the heart rate below sixty beats per minute. That could be normal for an athlete with a large heart (tennis champion Björn Borg's heart rate was reported to be thirty-five beats per minute), but it is abnormal for the majority of people. The vagus nerve has a branch to the heart, and manipulating it during surgery can inadvertently slow the heart—or even stop it.

"Do you want some glycopyrrolate?"

"Probably a good idea."

In fact, it was a very good idea and one I had not thought about. If the surgery did slow Emily's heart, that drug should block the effect.

"Central line?"

"No thanks."

A central line is a large-bore intravenous line (or multiple lines) usually placed in the jugular vein of the neck. It allows large volumes of fluid or blood to be given to a patient quickly. This can be life-saving when the patient is exsanguinating, but I had never needed to give a patient blood for this sort of operation. In fact, the procedure needed to be as bloodless as possible so I could see the small vessels and nerves.

"Art line?"

"Yup."

An arterial line is a special IV in an artery, not a vein. Usually in the radial artery of the wrist, it allows instant measurement of the blood pressure and can be used to draw blood for tests at any time.

"Foley?"

"I guess." A Foley catheter is placed through the urethra into the bladder during longer surgeries to drain urine.

"Anything else?"

"I need her P-A-C-O-2 hyperventilated down to 30 when I'm intradural."

Breathing quickly, hyperventilating, reduces the carbon dioxide concentration in your blood because you breathe out that gas, and reducing the carbon dioxide in the blood causes the blood vessels in the brain to constrict. When all of them constrict, they take up less space and the brain shrinks. Operating around a smaller brain inside the skull is always easier than trying to get around a larger brain plastered up against the inside of the skull. This trick to shrink the brain was used for decades before it was realized that aggressive hyperventilation, dramatically reducing the CO_2 level, could severely constrict the vessels and completely cut off the blood flow—causing deadly strokes. Eventually surgeons found a balance. My protocol was to hyperventilate the patient down to a P_aCO_2 of 30 mmHg (the normal measure of the carbon dioxide's pressure at sea level would be 40 millimetres of mercury, or mmHg). That typically shrank the brain enough to make it easier for me to work around it during the first part of the surgery.

It's likely that the manipulation of a brain's blood vessels through breathing techniques were recognized thousands of years ago by the yogic practice of the art of breathing, or *pranayama*. During a medical conference in Mumbai, I learned from a young yoga instructor that there are many different styles of breathing. I found the concept of "skull-shining" or *kapalabhati* especially interesting, because it is essentially aggressive hyperventilation to the point of dizziness. I wondered if this intense hyperventilation could cause localized ischemia (reduced blood supply causing brain dysfunction) in the region of the brain dealing with spatial awareness, which might make the yogi feel like they were floating, disconnected from earth or in another dimension.

Elinor had a series of other questions dealing with blood pressure parameters, diuretics, antibiotics, paralyzing agents and the type of anaesthesia. We went over all of them.

During this time, Betty had gowned and gloved and set up her sterile back table with most of the instruments we would need. Wai-Yee was handing her the sterile instrument sets in rectangular metal trays. She would hold each set with one hand beneath it, then unwrap it with the other, sequentially pulling its blue covers towards her arm and revealing the sterile tray inside like peeling a fruit. Betty then took the tray and set up the instruments on her table, which was covered with a light blue sterile drape, until the six-foot-long, two-foot-deep table was nearly covered. Wai-Yee announced she would get the patient.

My junior neurosurgical colleague, Dr. Peter Gooderham, pushed open the OR doors and leaned his head in. "When do you need me?"

"Patient's coming now, and I'll call you when we're intradural."

Peter was one of our residents who had completed his training and had recently come on staff. He was specializing in vascular neurosurgery, which deals with ruptured aneurysms and vascular malformations. It is the pinnacle of surgical dexterity and machismo.

Patients with ruptured aneurysms, a leaking blister on a blood vessel feeding their brain, usually need immediate surgery to place a titanium clip across that aneurysm to save their life. The surgery is urgent, difficult and high-stakes because the aneurysm is often deep at the base of the brain and requires a long dissection through a swollen brain to get there.

If the aneurysm bursts, the torrential arterial bleeding makes it impossible to see and likely fatal. If the clip does not completely close the aneurysm, the patient will likely die later of a hemorrhage. If the clip occludes the vessel harbouring the aneurysm, the resulting stroke can be devastating.

Vascular neurosurgeons are a different breed. At our weekly morbidity and mortality rounds, where we detail any complications from the week before, they could describe the patient who had died the day before during surgery from a horrendous complication and move on to the next case with an insignificant bladder infection without a pause. Life in the fast lane. I had clipped about one hundred aneurysms at the beginning of my career, but had not enjoyed any of them. After subspecializing in functional neurosurgery, I was only too happy to give up that part of my practice.

Peter was a surprisingly good surgeon for someone his age. At thirty-five, he was already technically gifted and had good judgment in patient selection. I'd wanted to be sure I was not completely out of line in offering Emily surgery, and Peter had agreed to review the case and provide a second opinion and to join me for the surgery. Usually our operations were the teaching grounds for our residents, our medical graduates specializing in neurosurgery. Throughout a six-year apprenticeship, the young doctors gradually assume more responsibilities during the operations. By the end of their training, they are supposed to be able to do the operation independently.

I found it difficult to allow someone with only a few years' experience to operate on my patients because I was responsible for their mistakes. If I were operating, it was far less likely mistakes would occur. Surgeons typically make mistakes at two moments in their career. In the early years, while they are still climbing up the learning curve, errors are made because they just do not know what to do. Late in their career, slip-ups occur because they are not paying attention. The involvement of neurosurgery residents increases the first type of mistake but reduces the second. Almost anyone can cut between two dangerous objects if they are paying attention, but how about one hundred times in a row? When a neurosurgeon stops focusing, or when the mundane repetition of an easy operation lures you into a complacent disinterest, complications follow.

The resident typically asks the question, "Why are you doing that?" even at the simplest point of the procedure. The fact that you need to teach someone the steps of an operation heightens your concentration and focuses you on the sequence of those steps. To have a young colleague such as Peter in the room magnified that advantage tenfold. He would be an asset, because the ultimate surgical assistant already knows the operation and is not learning it. They will know what you need to see and will retract tissues to allow it. They also know when to hold still, whereas newer residents are always moving to optimize their view.

Operating through a small hole deep inside the head is also dangerous under the microscope, because the assistant's hand movements can bang into yours and push your instrument into the brain. The microscope's magnified view makes the field of view (what you can actually see) small. You can see your instrument tip and the brain, but not your hands. Bringing a new instrument into the field of view is therefore difficult, because you rely on feel, not vision, to come back to the same spot. An inexperienced surgeon bangs around until they find the spot.

The OR doors were pushed open by Emily's stretcher. Wai-Yee introduced her.

"This is Emily Murphy and she is here for a right MVD. She is allergic to latex and has signed her consent."

Wai-Yee named everyone in the room, and Emily nodded for each name but did not look up. The stretcher was parked beside the Maquet table, and Wai-Yee stepped on the brake to lock it in place. Emily was encouraged to wiggle sideways onto the OR bed, which was covered with a yellow gel pad to soften lying on the firm plastic. The stretcher was wheeled out, and Emily lay on the OR bed feeling for the edges of the narrow table and adjusting her body to the middle.

We all paused for the time out, the second checklist from the WHO. Wai-Yee read out the patient's name and the operation listed on her consent form. Elinor confirmed she had no allergies to medications and her blood work was normal. I confirmed that all the equipment needed for the surgery was in the room and that I did not require any blood. We then introduced ourselves.

"I'm Chris. I'll be doing the operation."

"Peter. Assistant."

"Wai-Yee. Nurse."

"Betty. Nurse."

"Elinor. Anaesthesia."

"Henry. Anaesthesia resident."

"Felicity. Medical student." I had not noticed the medical student at the back of the room.

We were ready to go. Elinor took charge and guided Emily through the induction of anaesthetic. The next time I looked at Emily, she was fast sleep, with the endotracheal tube taped to her face. Her lines went in next. Wai-Yee placed a Foley catheter and Elinor's resident, Henry, put an art line in Emily's wrist.

"Call the movers," I said to Wai-Yee. She pressed the button on her Vocera, a voice activated paging system for OR personnel, and spoke slowly and clearly.

"Call Team 4 back."

Within a few minutes, the movers arrived—the people who helped move the patient into position for surgery.

We turned Emily onto her left side, legs bent at the hips and knees with pillows in between. Her left arm extended away from her body on a small arm board with a pillow to bend her elbow. Her right arm lay on her hip with a long Elastoplast tape pulling her right shoulder down towards her feet. Foam wrapped both her arms, both feet, and also her chest and back. A soft roll was slipped under her left upper chest to take the pressure off lying on her left arm.

"Hold her head," I told the smaller of the movers, who reached under her neck and picked her head off the headrest. I pulled the pillow out from under her head and dropped it on the floor to kneel on. Then I pulled the small headrest away from the main table, so her neck and head were now held in midair.

"Clamp," I said. I nodded to the other mover that I wanted the Mayfield headrest from the positioning table. I held the clamp with the single pin towards Emily's forehead and the double pins vertically oriented on her occiput (the back of her head). As I squeezed the clamp, it ratcheted together, clicking tighter as I squeezed. Peter injected local anaesthetic into the scalp where the three pins were. She was anaesthetized but the local reduced the need for additional general anaesthetic. The pins were pushed through her scalp into her skull, and I turned the screw until it showed three lines indicating sixty pounds of pressure.

I told the mover to let go. Holding the clamp, I positioned Emily's head, keeping her neck straight but flexing her head like a soldier looking at their feet. I rotated her head, so that she looked straight across the room. More rotation towards the floor would make it easier to look under the inside of the skull and around the outside of the brain, but it would also rotate the front of the brainstem away from me. I wanted to see the brainstem, where the vessel and nerve would be, even if it meant working harder to get there.

"Okay. Lock her in."

The mover sequentially tightened the screw linking the Mayfield clamp to its holder (its wrist), then the screw within the holder (its elbow), then the lever bracing the holder to the bed (its shoulder). The final lever closed with an audible thud that signalled I could let go. I reached up to Emily's head and tried to move it. It was rock steady.

I stood up and let the movers go.

"Shaver?" Peter handed me the electric shaver and I shaved a triangle of her hair straight back from the top of her right ear for two inches and then straight down to the nape of her neck. I like to put my incisions under the hairline, so they will be invisible in the future. A few locks of her black hair dropped to the ground and Wai-Yee scooped them up.

I put on sterile brown gloves and began scrubbing her scalp with a surgical brush filled with pink chlorhexidine. The brush foamed a pinkish lather that I used to mat down her hair. That first scrub was followed by two more using sponge cubes soaked with more of the pink stuff. After that, Peter and I left to scrub (wash our hands). I had planned to call him for the more delicate part of the surgery when we were "intradural," looking at the brain, but he had decided to stay for the whole case.

The scrub sink is a surgical sanctuary. There is a predictable moment before each case when you can pause and think. A moment to teach. A moment to talk. Somehow pleasurable, the routine reminds me of the approach on a diving board—always the same no matter how difficult the upcoming dive. Peter and I put on our loops and discussed the case.

"I think the compression will be near the brainstem," I said.

"Maybe, but we should look all the way out to the skull."

I agreed. There was not much more to say. I backed through the OR doors with my arms held up, still dripping water off my elbows. My loops were designed to focus at my working distance, my natural arm's reach, so the rest of the room was a blur. I looked over the top of the lenses to see everyone.

Betty handed me a green towel to dry my hands. She opened a gown and held it up so I could reach in both arms at once. Wai-Yee pulled the gown over my shoulders and tied it at the back. Betty opened my gloves and stretched the wrist open. I pushed my right hand in, then used it to help open the left wrist for my other hand. I double-glove. A study from Basel, Switzerland, showed that 15 percent of surgical gloves develop holes during surgery. Wearing two sets of gloves reduces the chance that any bacteria on your hand may contaminate the wound. The argument against this is the associated loss of feeling or touch through two gloves.

When I started operating, I always double-gloved so that I would learn what everything should feel like through two layers of 0.2 mm neoprene. There is a tradition in neurosurgery to triple-glove. We wear an extra glove when we place the drapes on the patient, and once they are completely covered, we remove the top glove.

I began by drawing a purple line behind Emily's right ear where we would make our incision, then covered the patient in a series of sterile blue drapes until all that could be seen of her was the purple line and less than an inch of skin on either side. I walked directly in front of her head with Peter on my right and Betty behind us. The nurse's back table was behind her with all our instruments.

The magnification of my loops was such that I could see only half of Emily's three-inch incision at one time. I put my left hand on the bottom of the purple line and reached back with my right towards Betty. She placed the scalpel in my fingers like a pencil before I asked for it. I paused long enough to ask, "Elinor, may I begin?"

"Yes. Thanks for asking," she replied, and I cut into Emily's skin along the length of the purple line.

The blade led, and my left thumb and index finger pulled the skin edges apart like a zipper as I went. Yellow bubbled fat beneath the skin appeared and small points of bleeding began. I rotated and reversed the direction of the knife blade and handed it back.

"Bipolar," I said aloud.

The bipolar is used to coagulate bleeding vessels by heating them with an electric current. Two thin, bayonet-shaped, blue metal blades extend like large tweezers, twice as long as your fingers, and are plugged into an electric cable at the other end. The current jumps from the tip of one blade to the other, cooking a few millimetres of tissue in between. The instrument was placed in my hand. I spot-welded all the small bleeders and continued.

Beneath the fat were several layers of muscles.

"Monopolar," I said. The instrument came as I spoke. The veteran scrub nurses knew the operations as well as I did.

The monopolar is a thin metal blade like a toothpick, extending from a plastic handle that is electrified when you press its yellow (cutting) or blue (coagulating) buttons. The monopolar hums when it is activated. Its grey plastic facade belies the importance of this instrument for surgery in general and neurosurgery in particular. Harvey Cushing first used the monopolar on October 1, 1926, to remove a particularly bloody brain tumour, which he had failed to remove three days earlier because of excessive bleeding. Cushing heard William Bovie describe his newly invented electrocautery device at rounds in the Peter Bent Brigham Hospital in Boston and asked if he could use it. The tumour was then removed "most satisfactorily" and the "Bovie" became an instant success. Older surgeons still call it the Bovie; most of the younger ones would not know what that is and call it a monopolar.

At this point, I cut down to Emily's skull and cleared all the muscles and tissues to the sides. A self-retaining retractor was inserted, which opened its teeth sideways and locked everything in place.

The skull is incredibly strong—pound for pound stronger than steel or concrete. On average, it takes over five hundred pounds to crush it. In contrast, your collarbone takes only seven. The juxtaposition of the strong skull and delicate brain requires extraordinary care when cutting through the skull to expose the brain.

Beneath Emily's skull bone was a layer of dura. This is a thick protective layer of connective tissue surrounding the brain and spinal cord. It is the outermost of three protective layers for the brain and takes its name, dura mater, indirectly from the Arabic for "tough mother." The mother of all protective layers. We owe a significant debt to our Arabic colleagues for their anatomical knowledge. As Europe slept during the Middle Ages, Persians and Arabs led the world in medicine. They translated the knowledge of the ancient Greeks into Arabic and then into Latin, where it became understandable for Western scholars.

I needed to cut through the dura to see the brain underneath. The potentially lethal complication at this moment would be to cut into the sigmoid venous sinus. The word "sinus," from the Latin "curve, fold or hollow," is more commonly associated with the nose, but in this case, the dura has a fold within it filled with blood. This large vascular channel inside the layers of the dura was at the edge of my exposure; it is where all the blood exiting from the brain pours down into the jugular vein in the neck. Bleeding from this structure would be torrential; the brain accepts a quarter of the body's blood flow from the heart.

Beneath the dura is the cerebellum, the "small brain" at the back of the head that controls coordination. Remarkably, there are more neurons in the cerebellum than its six-times-larger and evolutionarily newer partner, the cerebrum. The huge cerebrum provides a who's who of the functions necessary to be human—abstract thinking, planning, emotional control, language, movement and vision—whereas the cerebellum coordinates motor movement and is found in all vertebrates (and the octopus). Damaging it with my scalpel would damage the coordination of Emily's right arm.

In order to mentally visualize the orientation of these anatomical structures, you can cup your left hand around the fist of your right, like the passive Shaolin monk salute. The right side of the cerebellum is your right fist and the inside of the skull is your left fingers. I needed to see the brainstem, which would lie in front of your fist, where the tip of your right baby finger is. For this approach, we look under your left fingers and above the back of your right hand (or neurosurgically, inside the skull around the outside of the brain). Now let your fist fall away from your left fingers and you can begin to get the idea. Emily was lying on her side, so gravity would let her cerebellum fall away from the inside of her skull.

We had now reached the proverbial rock and a hard place of this operation.

The ideal place to cut the dura was over the far edge of the cerebellum; that way you can look around the brain without pulling on it. Unfortunately that is where the sigmoid venous sinus is located. The closer your dural cut to the sinus, the easier the next step of the procedure will be—looking around the edge of the cerebellum. But the more likely you are to get dangerous bleeding from the venous sinus. In contrast, the farther from the edge, the less likely for lethal bleeding, but you may damage the cerebellum by having to pull it too hard to see around it.

This is a moment for technical experience. The younger surgeon stops too short on their cut and relies on pulling the cerebellum to see around it. This is safe from bleeding, but the additional retraction causes brain swelling and closes off the viewing space. More pulling, more swelling. The surgery will later be described at rounds with the ubiquitous phrase, "It was harder than I thought." The more experienced surgeon will make the operation look easy. Cutting far out to the side of the dura, close to the sinus, allows a clear view around the corner of the cerebellum. A minimum of retraction, a clear view, and on to the next step.

I cut into Emily's dura with a long-handled scalpel. I scored the outer side of the leathery dura, then hooked the outer edge with a dural hook and pulled it up away from the brain and cut the rest of the way through. A small hole pierced the dura and air flowed in, allowing it to lift off the cerebellum. I then cut a semicircle in the dura the size of my thumbnail with the Metzenbaum scissors and sutured the flap up out of the way. This was the ideal opening size. I had discovered this years ago after an ill-advised period when I succumbed to the pure bravado of attempting smaller openings (the Japanese were describing dime-sized openings in the neurosurgical journals at the time).

With the dura open, a small portion of Emily's brain was now in full view. I could see, just as an ancient Egyptian had once described, "a pulsating structure with corrugated edges." It pulsed with the double rhythm of her heartbeat superimposed on her slow breathing. With each heartbeat, the brain quickly filled with blood and expanded slightly, then relaxed as the blood pressure dipped between beats. With each breath, the ventilator slowly pushed air into Emily's lungs, the rising pressure in her chest momentarily pushing back on the blood flowing out of her brain, down the sigmoid venous sinus and into her jugular veins. The brain slowly expanded outwards, engorged with blood in its veins, and pouted through the dural incision as the ventilator hissed air into her lungs.

On top of this slow, rolling wave of brain swelling with each breath were the smaller, quicker pulsations of the brain with each heartbeat. The brain then sank away as the ventilator exhaled for her, continuing with the smaller pulsations of each heartbeat.

I needed to see underneath the dura and above the brain. With the brain pouting through the dura, this was not possible. Elinor had hyperventilated Emily to shrink her brain, but it was not yet enough; I would need to drain cerebrospinal fluid. As we saw earlier, the brain (and spinal cord) floats in CSF, the water-like liquid that leaks from your ears after a bad skull fracture. It is the perfect growth medium for bacteria, and the resultant infection, meningitis, has a death rate of about 15 percent with antibiotics and 90 percent without. About five hundred people in the United States still die of meningitis each year.

Since the brain is floating in CSF, if it is drained, the brain will sink inside the skull, thereby opening up a view between the dura and brain. I began draining this fluid. I folded a half-inch cotton patty and pushed it between the dura and the brain, which allowed the CSF to slowly drain out while I set up for the intradural dissection. The brain replenishes its CSF several times a day.

"Drape the scope. Suctions to medium. Half-millimetre bipolar to 35. Give me the Greenberg." I spoke this list by rote.

Betty put a sterile drape around the microscope, and Wai-Yee reduced the strength of the suctions and bipolar.

The Greenberg is a retractor system that attaches to the Mayfield and allows me to rest my hands while operating. Everyone has a natural tremor, and it is magnified if you are operating from your shoulder and holding the instrument at the end of your arms. If you rest your hands on a metal bar, then the only tremor the instrument sees is from your fingers. This is essential when operating under the microscope because every movement is magnified.

I adjusted the retractors to rest my hypothenar eminences (the soft edge of the hands on the side of the little finger). The system also holds a self-retaining Sugita retractor, a thin, malleable, metal triangle. There are three sizes and, like Goldilocks found, the medium one is just right. When it is bent to the length of my index finger, it reaches inside the head far enough to touch the brainstem.

The microscope was wheeled towards us and locked in place. Wai-Yee took off my loops and put on my regular glasses. I grabbed the microscope handle and squeezed the finger trigger that allowed it to move freely. The two eyepieces had already been set to my interpupillary distance, and I adjusted the zoom and focused on the brain. Under the microscope, the brain is even more beautiful. It is whitish-pink, not grey, and the cerebellum has a rippled surface.

I removed the cotton patty, and there was a sliver of space between the inside of the dura and the outer surface of the brain. Patience was the key here; a hurried approach would mean pushing the cerebellum to look over it and that could tear a bridging vein still hidden beneath the dura. Eventually all the veins draining the brain must leave its surface and bridge across to the dura, where they enter the large venous sinuses I had taken care not to cut.

My approach to the trigeminal nerve is around the superior shoulder of the cerebellum in the groove where the tentorium attaches to the petrous bone. My approach to the vagus nerve today would be around the inferior shoulder of the cerebellum, similar to the approach to the facial nerve. Always up and around, or down and around, never just around. That can put too much tension on the eighth cranial nerve and cause permanent deafness.

The second protective covering of the brain is the arachnoid, named after the Latin word for spider because it looks like a spider's web. Usually transparent (unless scarred by meningitis), it has a beautiful gossamer appearance and tears easily to gain access beneath it. This layer covers the brain, like shrink-wrap, and is pulled over any vessel or nerve leaving it. As I looked around the lower corner of the cerebellum, the arachnoid curved around the brain, then turned up and over the lower cranial nerves, following them out to where they entered the inside of the skull. I increased the magnification and could see through the arachnoid.

Three nerves ultimately enter the skull through a small hole called the jugular foramen. The eleventh nerve (accessory) comes up from below because it originates from the upper spinal cord. The tenth nerve (vagus) begins as multiple little rootlets at the side of the brainstem that converge into one larger greyish nerve. The ninth (glossopharyngeal) nerve sits alone just above the vagus and is whiter and thicker than any of the vagus rootlets.

I cut through the arachnoid over these nerves with microscissors, and the nerves came sharply into view. I extended the arachnoid dissection up and over the eighth (vestibulocochlear) and seventh (facial) cranial nerves.

I asked for each instrument as I was finishing with the previous one.

"Number 9."

"Number 6."

"Rhoton scissors."

Instead, Betty handed me the Yaşargil scissors. It was what I wanted but could not ask for correctly.

"Number 6."

"Number . . ." I lost the number and held my finger up in a hook. Betty handed me the number 9. The surgeon's reduced ability to speak during surgery is a well-reported phenomenon. More precisely, it is described as a difficulty finding the right word. Some suggest that the intense focus on three-dimensional representation required by surgery, a function found in the parietal lobe, overwhelms the language function of the adjacent temporal lobe. Whatever the cause, the great nurses compensate. The old joke has the surgeon saying, "Hand me what I need, not what I asked for!"

Peter was looking through the other side of the microscope as we faced each other with Emily's brain between us.

"That must be it . . ." he said.

"Wow."

I was shocked. That really was it. The upper two of the six tiny nerve rootlets that joined together to form Emily's right vagus nerve were draped over a pulsating blood vessel and were being stretched severely. Everything I had wondered about, imagined and postulated was now in front of my eyes. I gazed at the anatomy and paused. The thin, thread-like rootlets were barely visible with the naked eye, but magnified by the microscope, they arched over the blood vessel like a bowstring pulled taught.

The choreographed dance of surgery came to a halt. The room went quiet. I looked at the rootlets in silent wonder. Betty held a small dissector in the air above my right hand, ready to give it to me, but I never asked for it. I just stared through the eyepiece.

This was the eureka moment for me. Emily had been trying to tell me something was wrong, and now I could see it. The truth lay exposed before me, and I just stared.

The pause may have lasted for a moment, or it could have been minutes. One's sense of time, like the fine control of speech, can also be lost during intense surgery.

Eventually Betty interjected, "Number 6 dissector?"

"Yes," I replied, but only after the instrument had already been placed in my hand.

I dissected along each of her vagus nerve rootlets. The lower four rootlets were completely normal. They gently curved down from their origin at the brainstem to their exit into the skull. The upper two rootlets, however, were bowed upwards, towards us peering in, like tight violin strings. They looked stuck together, and the first one was caught up against a loop of an arterial blood vessel.

I pressed the button on the microscope handle to videotape what we were seeing. I knew this was an important moment and I wanted to capture the anatomy.

"Look how tight those two rootlets are," Peter said.

"And the artery is pulsating against them," I added.

"That has got to be it."

"Yeah, I think so."

"What now?"

"I think we free them up."

The second rootlet looked like it was stuck to the first by a white condensation of arachnoid. The arachnoid was too tough to tear easily, so I sharply cut between the rootlet and the arachnoid scar. The second rootlet was released and it floated back down in line with the other, lower rootlets.

"Twang," Peter said.

The first rootlet presented a problem. It was caught up and draped over a blood vessel that made a loop behind the nerve, pushing it towards us and stretching it severely. The vessel then continued out, between the first and second rootlets, to pass above the lower rootlets and feed the brain.

I wanted to push the vessel loop backwards, away from us, to take the pressure off the first rootlet. Since the vessel continued to pass above the remaining lower rootlets, simply pushing the vessel backwards away from us would cause it to push down on the lower rootlets.

Another crossroads. Caught, like Odysseus, between the sea monsters Scylla and Charybdis.

Any damage to that vessel would cause a brainstem stroke that would possibly be fatal, most certainly debilitating. Cutting the first rootlet to completely free the vessel from it would cause permanent nerve damage; cutting and then reattaching the rootlet after freeing the vessel would be very high risk (and had never been done).

Eventually, we elected to rotate the curved loop of the vessel ninety degrees from its current position at right angles to the rootlets to one that was more parallel. The upper nerve rootlet relaxed back down into place, no longer tented up by the vessel loop. The vessel loop popped up towards us, no longer held down by the nerve rootlet. Now the vessel loop and the nerve rootlets lay beside each other in parallel and the pulsating vessel no longer hammered up against the nerve rootlets.

We proceeded to hold the vessel in place against the cerebellum with SURGICEL (cellulose cut to size) and TISSEEL (a fibrin glue).

I took a lot more pictures and videos.

"We're done," I announced to Elinor.

I looked over to Wai-Yee. "Put on the closing tunes."

Wai-Yee hit play. "Gimme Shelter" filled the room. Merry Clayton belted out her famous duet with Mick Jagger.

The tension dissipated in an instant. Everyone started talking about their weekend plans as we finished closing the hole in Emily's head.

8.

THE CURE

There was a brief moment of congratulations after Emily's operation, but little more than the acknowledgement of another successful brain surgery. Hours later, sitting at my office desk, looking out the window at Vancouver's lights, I wondered, *What the hell did I just find?*

The unique juxtaposition of Emily's vagus nerve and her posterior inferior cerebellar artery explained her unusual symptoms. The surgery to correct it was, thankfully, completed without complication. It remained to be seen whether her problem was solved, but I felt confident about the outcome.

And now the ramifications of what I had seen began to sink in. There must be hundreds of people with Emily's problem. Maybe thousands? This was the recognition of a new disease.

Then the doubts flooded in. How would I convince my colleagues this disease even existed? Why had it not been described before? How would I find these patients? Maybe this disease had been described before under another name. And if it hadn't, what name was I going to give it?

The naming of a new medical condition has changed styles over the years. Historically the disease might be given the name of the physician who discovered it or the place where it was discovered. James Parkinson (1755–1824) is the source of the name for Parkinson's disease, which he first wrote about in 1817. More recently, researchers use universal terms to describe new conditions. I would get to name this condition because I had discovered it.

The World Health Organization has put out guidelines for naming new human diseases (that I had not yet read at the time). They recommend that new human diseases not include place names (e.g., Spanish flu, German measles, or Wuhan virus) because it could engender racism. Some are still named for places—Ebola is a river in the Democratic Republic of Congo, and Lyme is a town in Connecticut. The WHO also does not like people's names, specific animals or scary adjectives associated with a disease.

Prion diseases, the world's most lethal diseases, with no cure and a 100 percent death rate, are a group that include fatal familial insomnia, Creutzfeldt-Jakob disease, kuru and mad cow disease. They break all the rules of naming. To be given the diagnosis of *fatal* familial insomnia must be truly frightening. Only kuru might be acceptable to the WHO, although the questionable circumstances around its discovery were certainly not. *Kuru* is the Fore word "to shake," one of the symptoms that preceded death in this isolated tribe in Papua New Guinea. The researcher who discovered the disease deduced that it was transmitted by the cannibalistic ritual of eating the brains of your dead enemies or relatives. He was lauded as a Nobel laureate but later reviled as an unrepentant pedophile. The mad cow disease outbreak in England had a similar mode of transmission, through animal feed contaminated with the brains of the beasts' fallen brethren.

Originally, I had looked for patients with unilateral contractions of their throat (choking). If a vessel pressing on the facial nerve could cause hemifacial spasm, then there should also be a condition in medicine to describe a vessel pressing on the vagus nerve resulting in hemi-throat contractions.

In medical terms, the throat is composed of the larynx and pharynx. Thus the name for Emily's condition should logically be hemi-laryngopharyngeal spasm. It did not take long to recognize an acronym could be comprised of the letters He.L.P.S., simplified down to HELPS. I had also thought about hemi *episodic* laryngopharyngeal spasm to emphasize the intermittent nature of the symptoms, but hemifacial spasm was also episodic and did not include that descriptor.

Emily Murphy had one more attack of choking the day after her surgery—then never again. At that time, neither of us knew if she was cured. As more time passed, though, it became clear that the operation had worked.

I saw her in my office six weeks after surgery to look at her wound and ask her about her symptoms. Emily said she felt normal for the first time in years and had had no more episodes of feeling her tongue was fat or choking—a sensation that had misled her physicians into thinking this was just an allergic reaction. She had been exposed to latex paint again after her surgery and it had not triggered any symptoms. It's likely that, in the past, the harsh fumes from the latex paint had triggered her choking, not an allergic reaction.

My plan was to wait a year to ensure her benefit was long-lasting and then publish her case report in the *Journal of Neurosurgery*. At our six-month and one-year post-op appointments, she was doing fine, and I finally found some free time to write the paper about two years after her surgery.

At this early stage of discovery, I only had Emily's case to consider when describing the typical symptoms of HELPS. I made two mistakes in generalizing her condition.

First, I had focused on her choking and her sensation of a fat tongue, but the latter sensation would turn out to be a rare symptom among the growing cohort of HELPS patients, not one of its core features. One small muscle in the tongue (palatoglossus) is innervated by the vagus, and over the following years only one other patient ever mentioned their tongue.

Second, I had ignored her coughing, instead focusing on the analogy between hemifacial spasm, a pure motor phenomenon, and HELPS. The vagus nerve has both motor and sensory branches (in fact, 80 percent of the nerve is sensory). The motor branches contract the muscles on one side of the throat, and the sensory branches sense touch on that side and trigger cough with a tickling sensation felt deep in the middle of the throat. Each new patient with HELPS reported both choking and coughing, and it soon became clear to me that coughing was also a core symptom.

There was another bump in the road while reporting Emily's case. After waiting more than a year to write the report, to ensure she was cured, I went to the microscope to upload the videos and pictures from her case—and they were gone. I was stunned with disbelief. We had three Pentero microscopes, and I checked all three but was unable to find the images from her surgery.

When I asked the charge nurse, she said the microscope I liked had been upgraded a month ago and there were no images on it that were more than a month old. I phoned Zeiss and asked if they could retrieve the file—without success.

One of my former patients worked for CSIS, the Canadian Security Intelligence Service. I called him and asked if he could pull the images off the microscope's hard drive after they had been deleted. He tried but the hard drive had been replaced, not merely deleted, during the upgrade.

Now what? How would I show my colleagues what I had seen?

I had always enjoyed drawing the brain; in fact, it was one of the first things that attracted me to neurosurgery. So I bought colouring pencils and drawing paper and made a series of drawings that depicted my impressions of the surgery. This was the best I could do.

When I submitted the manuscript to the *Journal of Neurosurgery*, all three reviewers felt the drawings were unacceptable and wondered why there were no photographs. The editor put it the most kindly: "We would be interested in seeing a revised version of the manuscript considering each of the points from the reviewers. You should provide photographs or a professional artist's illustration of the relevant anatomy."

At medical school in Toronto, we had shared an anatomy class with the students studying medical illustration, so I phoned my classmate Vicky Earle, who was now working in Vancouver as a medical illustrator. She was able to provide a series of beautiful, sophisticated illustrations within a week.

I submitted the revised manuscript together with Vicky's illustrations and the paper was accepted May 13, 2016. HELPS was now an officially recognized medical condition. It was a personal victory—I had always wanted to discover something new about the brain, and this would be my legacy. I also knew that there was someone, somewhere in the world, struggling to get medical professionals to believe that their choking and coughing was real. Now that someone had a chance.

I met with Dr. Morrison to discuss how to proceed after Emily's successful surgery. He had accumulated a series of patients over the years who had choking and coughing with no identifiable cause. Having had speech therapy, acid reflux therapy and psychotherapy with no benefit, they were now seeing Murray to get Botox to relieve their choking. Murray had become the maestro of that technique. He was the "throat botoxer" for the entire province.

When we sat down in his conference room at Vancouver General to make a list of potential patients, Leo Strait was at the top of that list. He was followed by six more people with similar symptoms.

We agreed that all of them should have an MRI to look at their vagus nerves—but MRIs were not quick to come by and, as we've seen, could take a year in our system. That necessitated a phone call to Dr. Manraj Heran, a neuroradiologist at the hospital who was also a friend of mine. A tall, handsome Indo-Canadian whose parents had immigrated to Prince Rupert, Raju, as everyone calls him, is the kind of doctor that you ask for help when a family member is sick or when there is a very difficult case you cannot figure out. I called him on his cell and soon enough our choking/coughing patients had their scans fast-tracked.

Leo had his surgery on July 5, 2016.

His symptoms were a bit different from Emily's. Whereas Emily had felt a circumferential squeeze, Leo could tell his left side was choking him. As we've seen, his choking was so severe he had had a tracheostomy. He'd been getting Botox injections from Murray every few months, which, although they had reduced the choking, had no effect on the coughing. Leo's coughing fits were so bad that he would see stars and have bad headaches afterwards.

It was the severity of Leo's coughing that made me pay attention to this symptom and confirm, in retrospect, that Emily had also had this problem. Leo's symptoms were left-sided and his MRI showed a curving vessel (the same posterior inferior cerebellar artery as with Emily) against his left vagus nerve, and so we were planning a left microvascular decompression.

Leo's surgery was different from Emily's. He was a big man, and everything is more difficult in large patients. Positioning bordered on the ludicrous, as the movers were less than a third his size.

My skin incision was curved to accommodate his thick skin and push it away from my visual corridor. The cleverest aspect of his surgery was how we were able to take advantage of his tracheostomy to intubate him. At my request, the anaesthesiologist placed his tube through Leo's tracheostomy, well below his throat and vocal cords, and straight into his trachea. I then asked the anaesthesiologist if he could use a bronchoscope to view Leo's throat and vocal cords while we did the surgery.

I planned to electrically stimulate each of the rootlets of the vagus nerve and videotape the effects on his throat. I hoped that Murray might have a videotape of Leo's throat during an attack and I could demonstrate that stimulating the compressed vagus rootlet with a nerve stimulator during surgery could exactly reproduce the same contractions. Unfortunately, Murray had never been able to get a video of Leo's attacks because they were intermittent, and of course, when they occurred, Leo felt like he was fighting for his life and did not want a laryngoscope down his throat.

The surgical approach around the bottom corner of the cerebellum was easier than it had been with Emily because Leo was older and had some brain atrophy. I dissected the arachnoid off the vagus nerve rootlets and could see the posterior inferior cerebellar artery, or PICA, pushing the lowest rootlet towards me. We spent more time than usual videotaping and photographing the operative view to gather proof.

I dissected between each of his six vagus rootlets to see between them and follow the vessel (initially hidden behind the nerve) heading up and then turning 180 degrees to head downwards. The curving vessel was caught against and pushing on the lowermost rootlet. I held the rootlets apart and sequentially photographed between all of them.

This would turn out to be a mistake. I would get beautiful pictures and videos of all aspects of the case, but the retraction of the rootlets would cause temporary dysfunction of his voice for two weeks and interfere with his ability to swallow for two months.

While the anaesthesiologist videotaped Leo's throat, I used a long blue nerve stimulator to activate each of his vagus nerve rootlets.

The rostral (closest to the top) rootlet caused no contractions. It must have been purely sensory. The same thing happened with rootlets numbers 2 and 3.

Rootlet number 4 caused a contraction of the left vocal cord.

Rootlet number 5 caused a contraction of the left vocal cord and throat directly above it.

Rootlet number 6 caused a pure left-sided throat contraction. It was this sixth rootlet that looked to be the most compressed by the blood vessel, so it fit that his symptoms were left-sided throat contractions.

Leo awoke in the recovery room and was then transferred to the neurosurgery intensive care unit. As soon as he was awake, he knew he was better. I asked how he was doing and he replied, "Great." But his voice was weak and breathy, like someone whispering. It was immediately obvious to me that I had injured the vagus nerve rootlets to his vocal cords. This was a serious complication, and my heart sunk as I smiled back at him. It would be unacceptable to trade choking for a paralyzed vocal cord. Had I pulled too hard on his vagus nerve rootlets? Not knowing how hard I could pull on those structures, I had gone over that proverbial edge in my desire to see his anatomy.

Later that night, when I was looking at the videos of the operation in my office, I backed them up on my office computer, the hospital server and a flash drive. I would not lose these images.

It then suddenly struck me why Emily could not attribute her choking to one side or the other, whereas Leo could. Emily probably had contractions of her vocal cords, whereas Leo had contractions of his throat. You cannot feel your vocal cords move—any contraction would likely be experienced as a generalized choking sensation. You can, however, feel your throat, and it's easy to feel if the left side or right side moves. The reported symptoms of HELPS must therefore depend on exactly which rootlets of the vagus nerve are affected.

I phoned Murray. We decided to wait a few days to see if the swelling of the nerve from my operative manipulations would subside. Leo was paying the price for my photographic ambition. In an attempt to get ideal pictures, I had pulled on the rootlets far too much.

The goal of the surgery was to decompress the nerve and allow it to heal so it would not fire intermittently, causing his symptoms. If the nerve was permanently damaged, his symptoms would also disappear because it could no longer fire. We do this all the time for trigeminal neuralgia, where we trade the patient's trigeminal pain for numbness in that region of the face. They get used to the numbness quite quickly, like white noise, and are happy as long as the nerve is numb. But when it heals from the numbness, the pain comes back. If Leo's resolution of symptoms was just because I had injured the nerve, like a huge dose of Botox, then his symptoms would return once the nerve healed sufficiently to fire again.

Leo's voice took two weeks to recover back to normal.

But we still had another problem. He could not swallow.

We put a nasogastric tube through Leo's nose into his stomach and fed him a liquid diet. Murray examined him and explained that the vagus nerve also controlled the muscular contractions of swallowing down the esophagus, propelling the food bolus towards the stomach. It then pulls the lower esophageal sphincter open, so the food can get into the stomach.

Leo's lower esophageal sphincter would not open. Whenever he tried swallowing food, he could feel it fall down his esophagus and get stuck. He had a very tough time with pills, so we switched all his medications to intravenous.

Leo spent two months on my ward with a feeding tube in his nose. He never complained once—he was not the complaining type. Leo was the salt of the earth. He could see I was upset with the complication and often perked me up with, "Hey Doc, the coughing is gone" or "The choking has gone, this is great, Doc."

At two months, we were contemplating gastric surgery to cut Leo's lower esophageal sphincter to facilitate his eating. Then he just started swallowing. The nerve had healed and was working again. I wondered if the choking and coughing would return as well, but it never did.

His symptoms never returned. Leo had his tracheostomy removed three months later.

———

Over the next two years, after our initial report about HELPS, we operated on another four patients with the condition—and two patients that I misdiagnosed with it. It was a steep learning curve. I learned as much from those mistakes as the successes and wrote several papers describing how best to diagnose and surgically cure HELPS. The last patient had coughing and choking triggered by any activity that raised her heart rate. She had spent the previous two years sleeping in her living room because the effort of climbing the stairs to her bedroom always triggered the coughing attacks. Six months after her surgery, she sent me a thank-you card with a picture of her hiking in Whistler.

When I received her card, I was recovering from hip surgery—which gave me a brief glimpse at being on the other side of the scalpel.

It was admittedly not a realistic glimpse; being a surgeon comes with certain benefits. The downsides of surgical life are well documented: overwork, divorce and mental health issues. The benefits are few but clear: a fascinating, helpful life and an inside scoop on the health system. I knew who should do my hip surgery, I knew who should do my anaesthesia, and my OR nurses rearranged their schedules to be there for my surgery.

I had damaged my left hip at twenty-six years old, when I was diving for the University of Toronto and practising twice a day. The repetitive deep left knee and hip bend during the hurdle approach to each dive eventually tore the labrum of my hip, the cartilage ring around the hip that provides cushioning and holds the joint together. After its seal was broken, my hip joint moved more than it should and caused the wear and tear of osteoarthritis over the years.

I remember having to switch my "hurdle" leg for diving at the time because it hurt so much. While I was studying in Oxford in the late 1980s, the English diving team let me train with them at Crystal Palace. I won the UK university diving championships on my wrong leg in 1987 and 1988. The competition was not nearly as strong as in Canada, but the experience did catch the attention of the Barbados Olympic committee, as I still held Barbadian citizenship. I have a bunch of great stories from those days of competitive diving, but I will recount only one.

In 1988 I competed for Barbados against Greg Louganis at the Seoul Olympics in the men's three-metre springboard diving championships. (Well, perhaps "competed" is too strong a word. It was more like I "participated." In those days there were still amateur participants at the Olympics.)

If you remember the movie *Amadeus,* you will know the story of Antonio Salieri, the Italian composer who was in Vienna at the same time as Mozart. Salieri was good enough to recognize Mozart's genius but never good enough to equal him. That would be me competing against the man we knew as Lougo. He was one of the few athletes who transcended his sport. In a sport where the winner was usually a few points ahead, Greg Louganis had won the 1984 Olympics by more than one hundred points. He was a Bob Beamon or a Jesse Owens.

During the ninth round of the men's preliminary event at the Jamsil Indoor Diving Pool on September 21, 1988, Lougo famously hit his head on the three-metre diving board. The next diver was already waiting on the ladder leading up to the board, and I was standing poolside, directly under the diving board, ready to follow him.

When I heard Lougo hit his head on the board, I hurried to the edge of the pool. I was going to jump in but could not yet see him through all the bubbles on the surface of the water. As soon as the bubbles cleared, he came to the surface. He looked okay. After my dive, a reverse two-and-a-half somersault tuck, I went over to his coach, Ron O'Brien, and asked if they needed any help suturing him. I had completed medical school and internship by then. To my surprise, he swore at me and told me to get the fuck away! They had all the help they needed. I moved along quickly and never thought about the incident again for many years.

It's likely Louganis's coach knew he was HIV positive at the time, and those were the days when we did not know how HIV and AIDS were transmitted. A few years later, people were still uncomfortable when Magic Johnson sweated near them on a basketball court, let alone bled on them. It was a time of fearing the unknown. I remember being scared as a young neurosurgeon operating on HIV-positive patients because we felt we were literally taking our lives in our hands.

In retrospect, I think Mr. O'Brien was probably just trying to protect me. No one knew much about HIV and AIDS at the time, and the fear of the unknown can be insurmountable. Now that we have learned more about this virus, it is less frightening. I am still very careful when operating on patients with HIV, but I'm not really scared any more. Contracting the virus from a patient would require a large bolus of blood to be injected into you, not just a nick from a scalpel. Knowledge has relegated the virus from the scourge of humanity to just another chronic illness.

My hip got me through those summer games, marathons on four continents, an Ironman, and the gold medal game of the World Masters Games Over-50 men's soccer tournament before it began to slowly reel me in. More about that game later. At this time I had met and surgically cured six patients with HELPS and had been fooled by similar symptoms in two other patients. I was beginning to understand what the common symptoms were—intermittent choking and coughing—and what the less common symptoms were—intermittent sensations of a fat tongue, hoarseness or loss of voice.

The diagnosis of any medical condition begins with a recognition of its pattern of symptoms. I thought I could recognize HELPS and, more importantly, I thought I could teach others how to recognize it. In the process of writing my observations down, something jumped out at me. A different pattern of symptoms causing a different disease. The discovery of VANCOUVER syndrome was about to happen.

9.

THE DISCOVERY OF
VANCOUVER SYNDROME

I had published our work on HELPS in the *Journal of Neurosurgery*. Now it was time to tell the world about this newly discovered condition.

After you've finished medical school, the field of medicine continues to advance. On the day of your graduation, you are up to date with all the relevant topics, but the very next day you start to fall behind. That goes for specialists too—you will continue to learn everything about your field until the day of your final fellowship examination, and then you carry that information with you as you practise for the rest of your life. To address the concern that physicians may lose that information later in life or be unaware of crucial new developments, various medical licensing colleges around the world have created Continuing Medical Education, or CME.

In the 1950s, CME took the form of teaching rounds or journal clubs, where physicians would discuss an informative case or a new article in a medical journal. During the 1960s, the pharmaceutical industry funded this process, and the topics and information were often presented in a biased fashion. Those were the days when doctors were invited to travel abroad, with all expenses paid by a pharmaceutical company, to listen to the latest information about a drug from that company. Equipped with information about only that product, and a personal financial benefit to using it, the doctors soon fell in line with the pharmaceutical company's agenda. Drugs were prescribed because they were associated with trips to Cancún, not because they had the best therapeutic profile.

There was a push-back against that type of biased CME by educational institutions and the more ethical physicians. Today physicians must prove they are keeping apprised of medical developments, and medical colleges scrutinize the types of activities that qualify as educational.

Nowadays the two most common means of CME are attending medical conferences and reading medical journals. My next task, following the journal publication, was to figure out at which conference to present HELPS.

I was planning to attend the World Society for Stereotactic and Functional Neurosurgery in Berlin in June 2017, so I submitted an abstract detailing my case series. It was accepted as a podium presentation. However, my oral presentation on HELPS in Berlin was given the last time slot on the last day of the meeting. Perhaps twenty people heard my talk, not exactly the turnout I was hoping for.

Earlier in the year, I had also applied to present our work at the second meeting of the World Neurosurgical Federation for Cranial Nerve Disorders. A Shanghai-based neurosurgeon had hosted the first meeting of this specialized group a year earlier in 2017. The attending neurosurgeons from around the world had a particular interest in microvascular decompression—the style of operation I had used for Emily and Leo. Decompressing the trigeminal nerve cures trigeminal neuralgia; decompressing the facial nerve cures hemifacial spasm; decompressing the glossopharyngeal nerve cures glossopharyngeal neuralgia; and now, I had evidence that decompressing the vagus could cure HELPS. If anyone needed to know about HELPS, it was this group of neurosurgeons, the ones who were experts in the MVD operation.

When I wrote the organizer and added that I was very interested in becoming part of this group, since I had an interest in MVD, the response was quick and favourable. In formal but slightly stilted English, the organizing committee asked me to provide two lectures at the meeting and also asked if I would consider being the next president of the society. That seemed a bit odd, until I read their bylaws, which stated that the president was responsible for hosting the meeting and for arranging travel and accommodation for the members of the board.

Somewhat mystified at the requirement, I said I would like to present at the meeting but could not be the president if it meant paying for everyone. A series of emails were exchanged, and I agreed I would "modernize" their bylaws and promote the society in North America and Europe. Now I needed to find a second topic to discuss besides HELPS. What else could I discuss?

At the very end of 2017, I had operated on a patient who had a combination of symptoms compatible with HELPS (choking and coughing) and glossopharyngeal neuralgia (electrical pain shooting down their left throat).

Glossopharyngeal neuralgia is a rare (1 in 1,000,000 people per year) but well-known condition. Unlike HELPS, which is painless, this type of neuralgia is excruciatingly painful, like a bolt of lightning or shards of glass radiating from your inner ear to deep down one side of your throat. Patients could always tell which side the pain was on, and it could be temporarily blocked by numbing the affected area. Historically physicians accomplished this by placing a cottonoid soaked in cocaine in the appropriate tonsillar fossa.

One cause of glossopharyngeal neuralgia is Eagle's syndrome, which is a well-known condition in ENT circles. Just after the ninth cranial nerve (the glossopharyngeal nerve) leaves the skull, where it travels through the upper neck to get to the throat, it can be stretched by an abnormally long styloid bone. The styloid bone juts down from the skull, pulled by the muscles that attach to it. Occasionally this bone gets too long and forces the nerve to bend around it. The constant rubbing of the nerve against the bone demyelinates the nerve (rubs off its insulation) and results in the vicious electrical pain of glossopharyngeal neuralgia.

In the old days, the treatment for Eagle's syndrome was as simple as it was brutal. The surgeon put their finger far back into the patient's mouth, felt for their styloid bone, and then pushed like hell until it broke.

Gagging, cracking, screaming.

With the nerve no longer stretched around the now broken bone, it healed and the painful bouts of glossopharyngeal neuralgia abated. Surgeons back in the day claimed there was never a recurrence, but one wonders whether, if there ever was one, patients might not tell their surgeons for fear of a repeat procedure. Nowadays, the surgical approach is more dignified but has the same goal—to decompress the nerve from rubbing on the bone.

My patient did not have Eagle's syndrome—a CT scan ruled out an abnormal styloid bone. An MRI showed that the cause of his neuralgia was a blood vessel pressing on the glossopharyngeal nerve near the brainstem.

What was particularly interesting about this case was the combination of symptoms. He had both glossopharyngeal neuralgia due to compression of the ninth cranial nerve *and* HELPS (choking and coughing) due to compression of his tenth cranial nerve (the vagus). These two nerves are very close together and exit the brainstem only a few millimetres apart.

During the surgery, I found one vessel pressing on both nerves. His glossopharyngeal throat pain resolved immediately, and his HELPS slowly resolved over the next six months. I decided to add that case report as my second lecture for the Shanghai meeting.

———

I arrived in Shanghai for the MVD meeting on a cold, clear day in January 2018. It was my second time in China in a year; I had been invited to Beijing University Hospital a few months earlier to talk about my work in deep brain stimulation.

In contrast to Vancouver, Shanghai is overwhelmingly large and densely populated, with no visible houses, just apartment blocks and high-rises. The conference was held in a hotel an hour north of Old Shanghai. Since it coincided with a local neurosurgical meeting, there were several hundred attendees.

I described the discovery of HELPS to a room full of neurosurgeons, showed my operative videos, and concluded with a video of Leo telling his story and describing how the surgery had saved him. It was like preaching to the converted. In contrast to the lecture in Berlin, this one felt immensely useful. Almost everyone who performed MVD in China was in the room, and they would be able to carry this new knowledge back to their surgical practices.

The glossopharyngeal neuralgia plus HELPS lecture followed, and several neurosurgeons asked if they could visit Vancouver to watch. I was standing at the elevator after the lectures, waiting to go up to my room, when a group of younger surgeons surrounded me and took turns taking selfies with me. When they had finished all the conceivable combinations of group photos, they each shook my hand, looked me in the eye and gave a thumbs-up. An unspoken approval that transcended culture and language. I think these surgeons had absorbed the knowledge that I had struggled to understand but had been happy to share. As I rode up the elevator, I found myself smiling and thinking about Emily and Leo. They should be the ones getting selfies with the next generation of surgeons. Their struggles will help future sufferers of HELPS around the globe.

The trappings of the conference were uniquely Chinese. The staff wore matching red outfits and were extraordinarily attentive. The banquet was beyond sumptuous, more like ostentatious, in its elaborate displays of a dizzying variety of food. We washed all of this down with glasses of Moutai and dozens of toasts. Moutai, which has been produced in the Guizhou Province for over two thousand years, is a clear alcohol—pure water, wheat and sorghum—as strong as whisky and just as expensive. The toast was *ganbei*, which means "dry cup," and so every round was a bottoms-up.

The banquet went late but the meeting started again first thing the next morning. Lectures from 7 a.m. to 7 p.m., and then another banquet. I slept on the flight home—exhausted from the meeting and too tired to be nervous. It had been a productive conference, a sharing of ideas between very different people with remarkably similar goals. The knowledge of HELPS would be spread across China, and I looked forward to hearing about their successful surgeries when I hosted the next meeting in Vancouver in two years' time. (That meeting would ultimately be postponed another two years because of COVID-19.)

The next meeting I attended was in Paris two months later. Unfortunately, the sixth edition of the International Conference on Otolaryngology turned out to be a complete waste of time. I had hoped to bring HELPS to the attention of my ENT colleagues, since they would be the ones who would likely see the patients first and need to make the diagnosis. Unbeknownst to me, the meeting was organized more as a vehicle for CME in a lovely location than a venue for learning. As I stood in front of the lectern staring out over a near-empty room, my colleagues were already up the Eiffel Tower.

In the first half of 2018, I attended the fourth annual Russian Federation of Stereotactic and Functional Neurosurgery meeting in Moscow to share my findings about HELPS at the invitation of the organizer. I travelled with my wife and our youngest, Max, and we were greeted at Sheremetyevo airport by the largest man I had ever met. He walked us to his car, sweating profusely and breathing hard. When he got in the driver's seat, his small four-door Scion tilted heavily. His belly pressed the steering wheel as we headed off for the ninety-minute drive into Moscow.

We were a block away from our hotel when he advanced into an intersection and slammed on the brakes to avoid a Mercedes G-class speeding right in front of us at over a hundred kilometres per hour. Looking over to my left, I saw this small tank of a car hurtling towards us, its engine revving. If our driver had not stopped, it would have been a speeding Mercedes versus a small car—I knew the result of that equation well. I might have survived due to the biggest human airbag between me and the car, but Karla, in the rear passenger seat, would not have. It was a sobering moment.

Our driver said something in Russian and pulled up to our hotel.

We stayed at the Holiday Inn Lesnaya for the meeting, which was well organized and attended by most of my Russian neurosurgical colleagues. I gave a plenary lecture, simultaneously translated into Russian, after a lovely introduction that highlighted the significance of the discovery of a new medical condition.

It was easy to get neurosurgeons excited about HELPS. It made sense to them, and they would be responsible for the operation to cure it. The meeting was successful; another part of the world now knew about HELPS. Unfortunately no ENT surgeons attended. If patients were going to be recognized and referred to my neurosurgical colleagues, I would also need to get the message to them.

After the meeting we moved to the Four Seasons on Red Square for two days of sightseeing in Moscow, joining the throngs that were walking around the huge square. The architecture of Lenin's Tomb reminded me of the tomb of Cyrus the Great in Iran, and Lenin's preserved body looked to me like a Madame Tussauds creation, though the official line was that it was still him. He looked perfectly lifelike, which seemed incompatible with our concierge's insight that his corpse had been eaten by fungus. A small group of scientists, called the mausoleum group, are responsible for maintaining Lenin's body (they also maintain Vietnam's Ho Chi Minh and the North Korean father-son duo Kim Il-sung and Kim Jong-il). Their work has moved away from preserving the actual biological tissue to preserving the look of the tissue; parts are therefore manufactured from plastic to look like a nose or a foot as needed.

When I returned to Vancouver, I was walking along Spanish Banks and thinking about writing up the case with the combined HELPS and glossopharyngeal neuralgia. It made sense because the ninth and tenth cranial nerves were so close together—why couldn't both be compressed by the same vessel?

That's when it all came together. If my HELPS patient could also have glossopharyngeal neuralgia, then why couldn't patients with glossopharyngeal neuralgia also have HELPS?

Glossopharyngeal neuralgia was first described in 1910 and there must have been hundreds of cases published over the century. Maybe one of them described additional symptoms compatible with HELPS?

Maybe we could find descriptions of HELPS from different countries or from a hundred years ago.

When I got to my office, I searched PubMed on my computer for all medical papers with the words "glossopharyngeal neuralgia" and found over a thousand. I refined the search to "reviews" and there were several hundred. I called our research team together and set out a plan. We would get every paper written on glossopharyngeal neuralgia and screen them for any symptoms of HELPS. My research coordinator could read Russian and Polish, and my fellows could read Spanish, German and French. We would try to find an example from each language.

Our efforts proved fruitful, uncovering several relevant cases:

- In 1948, the German neurosurgeon Gerhard Okonek described a seventy-year-old woman from Göttingen who presented with a history of left glossopharyngeal neuralgia. The painful attacks were followed by a dry cough (a symptom of HELPS). After dissection of the glossopharyngeal nerve, she had total relief of the pain and cough. The article was written in German, and thank goodness the case was recorded in 1948, after the Second World War. Earlier, after the First World War, German medical science almost completely disappeared when surgeons were banned from international meetings and the German language was banned from medical journals. Following the rise of the National Socialist Party in 1933, there was also a purge of German-Jewish surgeons from Germany, including Alice Rosenstein, perhaps the first female neurosurgeon in the world.

- In 1962, the Swedish neurosurgeon Einar Bohm published a paper while he was studying under the founder of Swedish neurosurgery, Herbert Olivecrona, at the Serafimer Hospital in Stockholm. Bohm would start the neurosurgery department in Uppsala the following year. His paper reviewed the thirty-year experience of eighteen patients with glossopharyngeal neuralgia in Stockholm, and two cases caught my eye. Case 11 "developed attacks of severe cramps in the throat, a feeling of suffocation and dyspnea." Case 14 "developed attacks of severe throat irritation which invariably led to protracted and severe coughing." These two patients were not cured with the standard sectioning of the glossopharyngeal nerve and only later had complete resolution of their symptoms when a few of the upper fibres of the vagus were cut during a second operation. Both described additional symptoms of HELPS.

- In 1972, the Argentinian head and neck surgeon Dr. Eugenio Borello wrote a paper in Spanish describing a patient with glossopharyngeal neuralgia and cough. The Russian physician Dr. M.N. Puzin wrote a similar paper in 1990.

- In 1981, the American neurologist Joseph G. Rushton reported the Mayo Clinic's experience with glossopharyngeal neuralgia from 1922 to 1977. Out of 217 patients, eighteen had an associated cough, two had loss of voice, and one had inspiratory stridor (closing of the throat when breathing in).

- In 1996, Dr. Anne-Laure Boch and her colleagues at the Groupe Hospitalier Pitié-Salpêtrière in Paris described a woman with paroxysmal and excruciating pain from the left ear to the throat (i.e., glossopharyngeal neuralgia) that would come four or five times and then be followed by cough. All her symptoms resolved following MVD.

The big picture for me was that HELPS had clearly been described (although not recognized) before and had occurred all over the world. Recognizing the symptoms in other cases in medical literature affirmed that it was not just a quirk of nature in a few patients in Vancouver. It was a real medical condition.

———

We were starting to get feedback from our earlier publications, and one question that came up was, Why were HELPS patients losing consciousness?

Glossopharyngeal neuralgia can have a rare (about 10 percent) association with an abnormal heart rhythm. When this occurs, the patient complains of swallowing-induced, one-sided electrical throat pain, and then their heart stops for a few seconds and they pass out. In my personal series of fourteen patients with surgery for glossopharyngeal neuralgia, I had one patient with this rare condition. His fascinating story not only contributes to our medical understanding, but also reveals the limited scope of the medical system when it comes to identifying unusual diseases.

The patient was a teacher from Victoria, the beautiful capital city of British Columbia at the southern tip of Vancouver Island. I had seen and operated on him more than ten years before. He developed left-sided intermittent and vicious throat pain several months after (and completely unrelated to) a cold for which his family practitioner prescribed a series of antibiotics that never worked. Each time he went to his doctor, he described the horrors of this intermittent pain, likening it to a searing hot poker being thrust through his ear and down his left throat. It usually happened after he swallowed a hot or a cold drink. Occasionally, after the blistering pain, he would pass out.

Each time the doctor saw nothing. The patient's throat looked completely normal. The chasm between the description of his symptoms and the reality of his examination concerned the doctor. He raised an eyebrow. Was the patient making this up? Was it a possible psychiatric manifestation?

On one visit, the teacher was so exasperated at the doctor's skepticism that he deliberately provoked an attack. He stood up, reached across the desk, picked up the doctor's coffee mug and drank a sip of the hot liquid. The swallowing triggered an attack and he grimaced in excruciating pain and then passed out, hitting his head on the corner of the doctor's desk and landing on the floor.

The doctor immediately called 911 and paramedics took the patient directly to the emergency department at the Royal Jubilee Hospital, where he was admitted and diagnosed with a heart rhythm problem that had caused him to faint. He had a pacemaker inserted by a cardiologist and was discharged the same day.

Just another day in the life of that cardiologist. When you are a hammer, everything looks like a nail.

The cruel irony for our teacher was that the pacemaker no longer allowed him to pass out. He was denied the blissful respite of unconsciousness. Modern medicine had condemned him to experience every agonizing moment of his pain.

Several colleagues had suggested the heart stopping for a few seconds might be the same mechanism by which our HELPS patients passed out. Others thought the choking might have been severe enough to cut off the oxygen supply and cause unconsciousness.

Our HELPS patients reported "fading out," not suddenly "passing out," which suggests their loss of consciousness was too slow for a cardiac rhythm problem. After reviewing the medical literature, our patients' fainting seemed more like the description of the medical condition cough syncope—and all our patients were coughing severely at the time.

Cough syncope was first well described by the French neurologist Jean-Martin Charcot in 1876. He called it "laryngeal vertigo." The rarer sneeze syncope and hiccup syncope would be described a hundred years later. Charcot, who has been called the "father of neurology," worked at the Salpêtrière Hospital in Paris and started the first neurology clinic in Europe in 1872. Originally a gunpowder factory (saltpetre being a component of gunpowder), the Salpêtrière facility was converted into a hospice for poor women in Paris in 1656 by Louis XIV, as well as a jail for prostitutes who were sometimes paired with convicts and sent to New France (Quebec). By the time of the French Revolution, it was the biggest hospital in the world. Now called the Groupe Hospitalier Pitié-Salpêtrière, it is where they tried to save Princess Diana's life following her tragic car accident.

Charcot was the first to describe many conditions, including multiple sclerosis, peroneal muscular atrophy and joint damage from diabetes, and he renamed *paralysis agitans* as Parkinson's disease. Some of the lustre of his career has been obscured by his focus on hysteria and claims about the benefit of hypnotism, which have been called into question in modern times. He did prophetically say, "To learn how to treat a disease, one must learn how to recognize it. The diagnosis is the best trump in the scheme of treatment."

The name "laryngeal vertigo" was changed to "tussive syncope" and eventually to "cough syncope" in the 1950s. The original mechanism, proposed by Charcot, was epilepsy—a coughing-induced seizure. Researchers in the 1980s used EEG (electroencephalogram) during attacks in several patients to rule this out. The focus then became the extreme cardiovascular changes during severe coughing, which resulted in decreased blood flow to the brain with resultant unconsciousness.

Pressure in the chest is extremely high during these coughing attacks, and various theories suggested that if the pressure in the chest is too high, then blood from the rest of the body trying to return to the heart cannot get inside the chest. The heart temporarily runs out of blood to pump up to the brain, and the patient faints.

Dr. Frederick Irving Knight, the first clinical professor of laryngology at Harvard Medical School, added to this theory. In 1886, Dr. Knight presented a paper criticizing Charcot's theory of laryngeal vertigo at the annual meeting of the American Laryngological Association. He argued that the loss of consciousness following coughing was not vertigo or epilepsy but rather syncope—a temporary drop in the amount of blood flowing to the brain. He summarized the world literature at the time with fourteen cases and added two of his own. "In four patients," he said, "there seems to have been decided evidence of a laryngeal spasm." Knight was describing severe episodes of choking and coughing leading to unconsciousness more than a hundred years ago. That *could* be HELPS if we were able to confirm it was one-sided, but it could also be any of the intermittent laryngeal obstructions such as vocal cord dysfunction (the term vocal fold is the more modern description of what we used to call the vocal cords—the name was changed because the structure is a fold of muscle of which only the inner edge vibrates rather than a cord strung between two ends). I knew that any of the historical descriptions of HELPS would be hidden inside similar descriptions of these more common two-sided problems. But what we needed was some way to tease out if any of these historical cases were one-sided, as is characteristic of glosso-pharyngeal neuralgia.

Our review had now found thirty-eight patients with glossopha-ryngeal neuralgia and additional symptoms compatible with HELPS. To our surprise, the distribution of those "additional symptoms" was not uniform. Whereas there were only four with the additional symp-toms of choking, thirty-three had the additional symptom of cough-ing. It was that unexpected finding—coughing and choking did not have to occur together—that led us to speculate about a completely new (unrecognized) medical condition.

Meanwhile, it took several more years before our teacher made it to us in Vancouver. Glossopharyngeal neuralgia is rare, but someone finally recognized the syndrome and referred him to us. An MVD operation cured his neuralgia and left him pain-free—with a now use-less pacemaker as a souvenir.

Just before my hip surgery in August 2018, I took my two fellows, Josue and Marie, hiking in Whistler, where the 2010 Winter Olympics were held. Our fellows are physicians who have qualified as neurosur-geons and are doing an extra year or two of subspecialization in func-tional neurosurgery.

We rode up the Whistler gondola to the top of the mountain, then hiked up and around the trail leading to the peak.

We were discussing the initial results of our search in the literature for patients with glossopharyngeal neuralgia and the additional symptoms of HELPS. What had become clear was that the additional two symptoms of coughing and choking seemed to be independently associated with glossopharyngeal neuralgia. In the literature over the last one hundred years, about 10 percent of patients with glossopharyngeal neuralgia had coughing, but only the rare patient had glossopharyngeal neuralgia with full-blown HELPS (choking and coughing). So what causes someone with glossopharyngeal neuralgia to *also* have coughing?

I postulated that if the nerve fibres to the throat transmitting sharp pain are affected, the result will be the typical swallow-induced sharp pain on one side of the throat (that is, pure glossopharyngeal neuralgia). If the nerve fibres involved are carrying sensation below that (to the larynx, trachea or lungs), then there will also be cough. The nerves to the larynx and trachea do not provide sharp pain, they just send a sensation like a tickle back to the brain, which triggers reflexive coughing.

When a child aspirates a coin into their lungs, they do not feel pain—they just cough. But when they swallow a fish bone and it gets stuck in their throat, it hurts. Why can you feel sharp pain in your throat but not below your throat?

Perhaps it was an evolutionary advantage to have sharp pain in the throat so you knew where to pull out that fish bone? If the fish bone got lower into your trachea, you would never be able to pull it out. The ability to feel the fish bone sharply on one side of your trachea would be unnecessary and perhaps debilitating. What you would need to survive would be for that fishbone to trigger a cough until it was dislodged.

Humans developed an elongated throat around one hundred thousand years ago. Our more ape-like ancestors before that, *Homo erectus*, had a very short throat between the back of their mouth and the top of their larynx. The descent of the human larynx and resultant longer throat came with a disadvantage—choking when eating. That disadvantage was overwhelmed by a tremendous new advantage—speech. Humans can speak, whereas chimpanzees can only vocalize. In the early 1960s, many scientists tried to teach chimpanzees to speak (coincidental with the space program), but no one was ever successful.

Primatologists such as Jane Goodall, as well as Allen and Beatrix Gardner, have taught us that chimpanzees can learn some sign language, use tools, feel empathy and remorse, and have a complex social structure. They just do not have the anatomy to be able to speak. When our ancestors, *Homo sapiens*, developed the ability to speak with their elongated throat, the evolutionary advantage must have been spectacular. They could coordinate attacks in the dark and at a distance. Choking was a small price to pay for the success of our species.

What suddenly struck me, as we were trudging up the steep gravel road of Pika's Traverse, was the concept that a patient could have a vascular compression cause them either pure glossopharyngeal neuralgia or glossopharyngeal neuralgia and coughing—depending on the local anatomy of the compression.

If that was true, why couldn't you have a vascular compression just cause a cough?

I postulated that the nerve fibres affected in this theoretical disease would not be the glossopharyngeal (since they cause pain), but rather—just below them—the most superior fibres of the vagus nerve. We had stimulated those upper fibres in Leo and our other previous cases and seen no muscular contraction in response. They must have a sensory function. Perhaps they are sensory fibres to the lower respiratory tract (larynx, trachea and lungs) that trigger cough when activated.

I wondered if a vascular compression of the sensory component of the vagus nerve would cause a neurogenic cough.

As we sat in the Rendezvous Lodge over coffee, we discussed, in fun, what we would call this condition. It didn't take us long to come up with Vagus Associated Neurogenic Cough Occurring due to Unilateral Vascular Encroachment of its Rootlet.

Hmm. Yikes. A mouthful and a half.

But the acronym that emerged from it was irresistible. Whether we could proceed to prove it existed or not, VANCOUVER syndrome entered our day-to-day lexicon. We had a new condition, and I thought Dr. Morrison probably had a few patients.

I called Murray and he sent the first patient to my office. A gentleman with unexplained cough and an MRI showing a large vessel distorting his left vagus nerve. Armando would also be one of the most delightful patients I had ever met.

10.

ARMANDO'S DELIGHT

Armando Arantes was a sixty-year-old man from Foz do Iguaçu, a border town between Argentina and Brazil. He was delighted to discover I had visited his hometown, mainly to see the spectacular waterfall that film buffs might recall as the focal point of the 1986 movie *The Mission*.

Armando had moved to Canada as a young man and had brought his Latin accent and gusto for life with him. He was an ebullient character, yet he always spoke softly, almost whispering as if he was telling you a secret, but accompanied by exaggerated facial expressions and hand gesticulations—seemingly to make up for the quietness. The combination sometimes made him seem comical. I liked him very much. I soon learned there was a medical cause for his strange manner of communicating.

Armando had a fifteen-year history of a dry cough. He described it as an uncontrollable response to a tickling sensation deep in his throat, just behind his Adam's apple. The coughing fits would occur throughout the day, and occasionally they were so severe he felt like he might pass out. After more than a decade of trying to quell the symptom, no medication had worked. His coughing continued spontaneously, but he could aggravate it if he was not careful.

I asked him what made his cough worse.

"What doesn't, Doc?" he whispered.

We then proceeded to have one of the more memorable exchanges I've ever had with a patient.

"I'll tell you what really gets it going," Armando said, confidentially but also somewhat teasingly. "Singing and sex!"

"What?"

"Anytime I raise my voice or sing . . ." he began.

The singing did not interest me.

"No. The sex part."

I leaned forwards to hear him better.

"Oh, Doc," he said. It was hard to tell whether Armando was going to become forlorn or nostalgic. Or if he was imitating a gangster in some black and white movie.

"When I'm with a woman . . ."

I nodded.

Armando was seated to my left, beside my desk. He leaned closer to me, as if there were other people in my small office.

"As I'm finishing . . ."

In order to speak sideways to me, as if in secret, Armando held up the back of his left hand to the right side of his face, shielding his lips, to whisper in confidence. A bit like Groucho Marx used to do. Perhaps there was a punchline coming.

". . . I always yell out—and then the damn coughing starts!"

I wasn't sure how to respond. Should I commiserate or cheer?

"Every time!"

I knew this wasn't supposed to be funny, but at the same time it seemed like it could be a vaudeville joke.

"*Feliz y triste,*" Armando whispered.

As I listened to this tale of lamentable ecstasy, I could not help but wonder how this Latin lover's partners might respond. Did Armando give them advance notice? It was difficult to regain my professional aplomb, but just as Emily's symptoms suggested to me she was suffering from HELPS, Armando's description of his ailment indicated he might have VANCOUVER syndrome. In fact, he would be the first person in the world recognized with this condition.

It certainly changed the mood. I explained to Armando that part of the vagus nerve normally sends a tickling sensation from deep in the throat when any object is lodged there. In his case there was no object, but because the nerve was firing spontaneously, it felt like there was.

"It's just like the tingling in your hand when you hit your funny bone," I said. "When that happens, there's no problem in your hand, you have just banged the nerve that comes from your hand as it passes by the elbow. Your brain does not know why the nerve fired, it just feels the sensations that particular nerve carries—tingling in the hand."

If Armando's nerve was short-circuiting and firing inappropriately, then medications to quiet the nerve should help. We use these medications (such as Carbamazepine) all the time for trigeminal neuralgia, where the short-circuiting of the trigeminal nerve causes bolts of lightning pain to shoot through the face.

Armando agreed to try Carbamazepine. I put him on a small dose, and he showed a remarkable improvement in his cough over the next few weeks. At best, he reported his cough was 80 percent better, although it was never completely gone. I was going to titrate up this medication, but he had a rare side effect—suicidal ideation.

In January 2008, the US Food and Drug Administration (FDA) issued a warning to healthcare professionals about the potential for an increased risk of suicidal thinking and behaviour associated with anti-epileptic drugs. The risk factor was 0.4 percent, so approximately four in one thousand patients taking the drugs. The general population has a 0.2 percent risk of suicide. Those taking the drugs are therefore twice as likely to attempt suicide (although it is still rare).

I stopped the Carbamazepine, and within a week his coughing returned to its previous full extent. We could not risk a different anti-epileptic drug, and so surgery became a possibility. Armando had a cough and a large vessel curving into and distorting his left vagus nerve. I had operated on Emily, Leo and a half-dozen patients with HELPS, but this was a different condition.

Once again, we needed a definitive test.

I extended the analogy of trigeminal neuralgia a bit further. In that condition, if you make one side of the face numb, the pain stops. In fact, that works so well that there is a common operation I do called trigeminal rhizotomy, where the nerve is deliberately damaged by heat to cause years of numbness and resultant pain relief.

If we could make one side of his throat numb and the coughing stopped, that would be a very good predictor of surgical success. Particularly if you made the other side numb and it didn't stop the coughing.

I talked to the new doctor who had now taken over Dr. Morrison's practice, Dr. Amanda Hu, about the practicalities of the numbing procedure. The devil is always in the details.

Hu explained that the numbness would have to be far more extensive than just the throat. In fact, the actual throat was probably not involved, because the sensation felt there was sharp and not a tickle. Below the throat, cough could be triggered by vagus nerve stimulation from the larynx, trachea and each bronchus leading deep into the two lungs.

Research has shown cough can be triggered by either stimulation of a mechanoreceptor or a nociceptor. The mechanoreceptors sense touch and are located in the larynx, trachea and bronchi leading to the lungs. They trigger if a foreign object is approaching the lungs. The nociceptors sense inflammation or noxious chemicals and are located deeper in the lungs. They trigger when a noxious chemical (such as capsaicin from bear spray) is in the lungs. All these receptors send their signals to the brain along the vagus nerve, which enters the brain and relays in the "cough centre" of the nucleus tractus solitarius.

How were we going to anaesthetize one side of the larynx, trachea and lung?

With thanks to Sir Victor Horsley, the nerve supply to the upper airway (larynx) is well known. The vagus nerve splits into many smaller nerves, including the superior and recurrent laryngeal nerves. The superior has an internal portion that provides sensation just above the vocal cords, and the recurrent provides sensation below the level of the cords and part of the upper trachea. Dr. Hu said it would be a routine test to anaesthetize the superior laryngeal nerve with some local anaesthetic. Routine for her, but still a needle through the throat for our patient.

It would be very difficult to anaesthetize one half of the lower airway (trachea, bronchi and deep into one lung). I wondered about intubating the patient and then squirting local anaesthetic down the tube, with the patient lying on one side. Would the anaesthetic preferentially drip down and cover the lower side? Our anaesthesiologists said this would not work because the spray would go everywhere. What about the double tube that is used when one lung is deliberately deflated for surgery and the other lung is kept inflated for ventilation—could you inject aerosolized local anaesthetic through one of the tubes? That seemed complex.

Our best chance was with the routine local anaesthetic block of the superior laryngeal nerve. Hu saw Armando in her office and anaesthetized his left larynx, but there was no change in his coughing. He returned two weeks later to have the other side anaesthetized. Again there was no change. Now what?

And so it was that I called Armando back to my office and presented all the information and my thoughts. To my surprise, he did not hesitate. He wanted the chance to be cured, even if it was just a chance. I presented the potential risks. He acknowledged them, signed the surgical consent form and asked when the surgery would be.

It was in the fall of 2018.

The operation was not difficult. When I came around the lower corner of the cerebellum and looked at the lower cranial nerves, I could see the blood vessel pushing on his vagus nerve rootlets. The curve of the vessel was pushing it into the vagus nerve and the arachnoid adhesions were holding the nerve rootlets from getting out of the way. Once I had freed up the tethering arachnoid bands, the nerve rootlets were pushed aside, and the vessel popped out at me. I deflected it away from the vagus nerve and kept it there with some padding and glue.

After the surgery, Armando had a coughing fit in the recovery room, and then never again. The tickling sensation that triggered his cough was gone.

I went to see him the next day. As I came off the elevator and walked around the corner towards the doors to the ward, I could hear singing. That was very unusual for a neurosurgery intensive care ward. Most of our patients are sedated with medications or by their own brain dysfunction. Occasionally there is yelling. Damage to the frontal lobes releases a thousand years of civilization's inhibitions and erases everything you ever learned in kindergarten. Patients who are disinhibited will say, yell or do whatever comes into their minds.

Singing was different. Surprisingly pleasant and equally intriguing. Who was singing and why? I pushed through the doors and the lyrics of "O sole mio" became clear. All the nurses around the front

177

desk turned and looked at me. Everyone was smiling. The charge nurse rushed up to me.

"Mr. Arantes has been singing all morning, Doctor."

"Is he good?" I joked.

"Yes, Doctor."

I continued to his room. Armando was sitting up in bed singing. One hand was on his chest, the other extended outwards, Pavarotti-like, reaching towards his imaginary audience. He stopped when I entered.

"Doctor, do you remember those two things I told you that always made me cough?" he asked, raising his eyebrows up and down.

I smiled and nodded.

"Doctor, I have been singing all morning with no coughing!"

Then, in classic Armando style, he held his hand upright, to the side of his mouth again, the way he had done in my office when we met the first time, but no longer whispering.

"I can't wait to try the other thing!"

———

I saw Armando in follow-up at six weeks, six months and then at one year—there was no more coughing. We published the case report, and VANCOUVER syndrome entered the medical world as an officially recognized, new medical condition on December 1, 2019.

I would not have discovered HELPS and VANCOUVER syndrome without Emily, Leo and Armando. There were a number of other patients whose individual stories and success or failure following surgery crystallized my understanding of these conditions. Each of them had refused to be ignored and had pushed for a solution to their problem. Each of them had fought against being dismissed by the medical system. Each of them had been unlucky to have an unknown illness, but lucky to live at a time and in a society where they could be their own patient advocates. Their struggles were personally successful and they had also cleared a path for other patients around the world.

I wonder how many others have been incorrectly convinced "it's all in your head." All of the patients with HELPS that I have operated on were told at one point that their condition was psychiatric. Of course, the stress of living with a condition that causes unpredictable choking and coughing to the point of unconsciousness would make anyone anxious. Avoiding all the foods, smells or activities that happened to occur before a previous attack would make anyone appear obsessive-compulsive. Continuously being told your physical condition was just psychological would make anyone angry. And having the courage to tell your doctor that they must be wrong would get anyone labelled as difficult.

Emily, in particular, refused to give up trying to find out what was the matter with her throat. She forced me to think beyond my training and imagine there was another possible cause for her condition, one that I had considered but never encountered. Her six-year struggle to get a three-hour operation was an ordeal, but she told me the result was a miracle.

The word "miracle" is too easily used in the medical world. Emily's success was a mixture of perseverance, hard work and thoughtful consideration. Real miracles are very rare. I have only witnessed two. The next story, about Nadia, recounts one of them and still leaves me full of wonder.

11.

NADIA'S MIRACLE

A miracle is often defined as a surprising and welcomed event that cannot be explained by natural or scientific laws and is therefore considered to be the work of a divine agency.

As our understanding of the world increases, what once may have been considered a miracle can often now be explained by science. His Liberian family may have thought it a miracle that Luogon Ouamouno walked out of the Tappita hospital, but, exposed to a few decades of neurosurgical practice and numerous similar cases, they would have been more likely to see it as a matter of course.

Miracles, the basis for sainthood in the Catholic Church, almost always involve an unexpected medical cure. To be canonized as a saint, a deceased person must perform two miracles (it used to be three, before John Paul II lowered the bar for everyone). If someone has an incurable condition and they pray directly (and only) to a saintly candidate, their subsequent cure proves that the candidate heard them and spoke to God on their behalf. This direct access to God and his divine cure proves saintliness.

The Vatican has a miracle commission, the Congregation for the Causes of Saints, which adjudicates each claim. There are three levels of miracles. Resurrection from the dead is the first and, as you can imagine, is not often evoked these days. A cure of the incurable is the second level. An unexpectedly rapid cure of a curable disease is the third. As science improves and the unexplained cures are reduced, the Church may revert to its pre-1531 position that miracles are not required for sainthood—only the demonstration of a holy life lived.

Pope John Paul II certainly lived a holy life and warranted sainthood. He was canonized on September 30, 2013, just eight years after his death. His reported miracles, however, have raised some eyebrows. His first posthumous miracle (the first one gets you beatified, the second sainthood) was a French nun with reported Parkinson's disease who said she was cured after praying to the former pontiff, who had suffered with the same condition towards the end of his life.

The nun's miraculous recovery was questioned because she later succumbed to the condition again and the diagnosis is always difficult to confirm before death. John Paul II's second miracle followed the cure of a Costa Rican lawyer with an inoperable brain aneurysm that disappeared after she prayed to him. Certainly rare, but miraculous? The Catholic neurosurgeon who reported he had never seen this before presented the case to his Latin American colleagues, and they were equally impressed.

There are many previous miracles that can now be explained by science. Today, a virgin birth (Matthew 1:18–25) is not unusual following the popularization of artificial insemination. Curing the lame is a daily routine in some hospitals, although not performed as spectacularly as by St. Peter (Acts 3:1–11). Curing the blind (Mark 8:22–26) can be done in a fifteen-minute operation performed by nurses (as I discovered in Liberia) and ophthalmologists.

Scientists are taught to question miracles. To debunk them. To search for an explanation. Religious leaders are taught to embrace them. To accept them. To be comfortable that faith can explain them.

Faith, the unquestioning belief that does not require explanation, is the antithesis of science. Many scientists, however, still believe in miracles. Professor Jacalyn Duffin wrote a book examining the Vatican sources documenting over 1,400 miracles (more than 90 percent were medical) and concluded that miracles exist.

I agree. Nadia Daly's cure is a phenomenon I witnessed but cannot explain. As science progresses, I hope the cause may one day become clear. We are actively investigating this case in the hope that it will lead to a new understanding and treatment for chronic pain.

The story begins in Edmonton, Alberta, in early 1982, although I would not meet the patient for another two decades. Nadia was a thirty-two-year-old woman working as a primary school teacher. One evening, while eating dinner with her husband, Charles, she bit down hard on some crusted bread and noticed a sudden shot of sharp pain from her back teeth on the right side. She washed the food out of her mouth with a sip of ice water, and the pain hit her again, causing her to wince and reach for her jaw. The pain was gone just as fast. Something was definitely wrong with her teeth.

Nadia phoned her dentist the next morning and was booked for an appointment a week later. During that week, the pain came and went. When it came, she could not tolerate any hot or cold liquids near the area. She was careful to drink just on the left side of her mouth and completely avoided ice water. Biting was sometimes possible, but at other times it triggered a sharp, stabbing discomfort. She had localized the pain to her back lower molars on the right side.

Her dentist examined her and diagnosed a crack extending into the pulp of the tooth just in front of her last lower right molar. With the crack extending into the pulp, she was told she would need a root canal.

That root canal would be her undoing. It would change every aspect of her life, her work and her marriage.

Nadia's dentist did not perform root canals, so she was referred to a colleague who was an endodontist. The endodontist would clean out the inner pulp of her tooth and temporarily cap it, then she would return to her dentist to have a crown placed on the tooth to hold it together permanently.

The endodontist had a very busy practice, and Nadia's procedure was booked for two weeks later. He would do five root canals that day; Nadia would be the last. The procedure began with a local anaesthetic to numb her lower right teeth. Nadia felt the sharp prick of the needle at the very back of her lower gum.

The treatment of dental pain dates to Babylon (2500 BCE), where physicians used a mixture of henbane, which contains the pain-killing alkaloid hyoscine, and gum mastic, the antibacterial resin from a pistachio tree, to soothe their patients. The first use of a local anaesthetic during dentistry followed Dr. Karl Koller's discovery of the anaesthetic properties of cocaine in 1884. Koller, who worked in Vienna as an ophthalmologist, was a colleague of Sigmund Freud.

Freud and Koller worked together studying the systemic effects of cocaine. They received a free and steady supply from the pharmaceutical companies Pfizer and Merck. They tested the drug on themselves, and in a paper, Freud extolled its "gorgeous excitement." Koller had searched unsuccessfully for many years for a local anaesthetic that could be used for eye surgery. After noting that the direct application of cocaine to his tongue made it numb, he realized that it might be just what he had been looking for. He tested topical cocaine on animals, then himself, then his patients. Within four years, it was being used for eye surgery around the world. After Koller died, a reprint of one of the papers he had written with Freud was found in his office with the dedication from Freud, to his "dear friend Coca Koller." Koller's technique was soon widely adopted by dentists, but as cocaine proved highly addictive, lidocaine has gradually replaced it over the last fifty years as the local anaesthetic of choice.

When Nadia Daly's endodontist returned a few minutes later, her right lower jaw was frozen; her tongue and lower lip were numb and felt fat and swollen. The endodontist began the work of drilling into her tooth and reaming out its inner pulp. Nadia could feel a deep discomfort during the drilling, causing her to wince and try to pull her head back. The endodontist paused and removed the drill.

"A bit more local will help," he reassured her.

The endodontist loaded another vial of lidocaine into a syringe and pulled back the corner of Nadia's mouth to reach the back of her jaw. Nadia did not feel the needle, just some pressure. "Back in a second," he said as he left the room again.

Nadia wondered whether he might use laughing gas. She had never had any but thought it was used during bigger dental procedures.

Prior to local anaesthetics, dental procedures could be done under the influence of either nitrous oxide, colloquially known as laughing gas, or ether. After painlessly extracting a tooth with the aid of an ether-soaked handkerchief, Harvard dentist Dr. William Morton was famously asked to demonstrate the technique for a bigger operation. He provided what has come to be known as the first general anaesthetic during an operation to remove a neck tumour at Massachusetts General Hospital in 1846. Dr. Morton spent the rest of his life trying, unsuccessfully, to patent the procedure and profit from his discovery. His colleagues and the public derided him for his apparent greed in the face of such an important discovery that could help so many.

Nadia's endodontist returned and began drilling again. She immediately felt discomfort again, squirmed and pulled away. The endodontist stopped. "You're really sensitive," he remarked. "I'll give you a bit more."

As he injected the local, Nadia felt a lightning bolt of pain flash through the right side of her face—as if electricity from a live wire had been stuck into her jaw. It was excruciating. She screamed, gripped the handles of her chair and lifted her body up like a board. After a few seconds, she relaxed back down into the chair. Neither of them realized that the needle and anaesthetic had gone directly into the nerve—permanently damaging it—instead of just beside the nerve to numb it.

"Oh my God. What was that?" she asked, her voice muffled by the bite block that kept her jaw open.

"Wow, you're very sensitive," the endodontist replied.

Nadia thought it must be her fault because she was "sensitive." She was still a bit fuzzy from the blistering intensity of the pain, but the discomfort soon settled. Holding on tightly to the armrests, she sat back further into the chair. She started to cry but kept still.

The drilling continued. She could feel its vibrations and smelled an odour like that of burnt hair, but it no longer hurt. Nadia lost track of time and any of the details of the rest of the procedure. When it was eventually over, her husband came to get her, and she left feeling nauseous and completely exhausted. They were home within an hour; her face was still numb and felt hugely swollen, although when she checked in the mirror it looked surprisingly normal.

A few hours later, the pain began.

Initially, a dull throb grew in her lower right jaw as the anaesthetic was wearing off. The sensation that her tongue was fat was fading, but the pain in her jaw was ramping up. Over the next six hours, Nadia would experience a degree of pain she had never imagined possible. It slowly but relentlessly escalated, each hour reaching a new level she had never experienced, only to be surpassed in the next hour. She had given birth, but this was worse in an uncontrolled and unexpected way. She also felt alone. When she'd given birth, she was surrounded by a small team of supporters encouraging her forward towards expected relief. Now her husband was with her, but he had no idea how to reassure her. He left to get the pain pills the endodontist had prescribed.

Nadia was now physically and emotionally alone. She paced in the kitchen. She pulled out a zip-lock bag, filled it with ice and held it against her jaw, then continued to pace, not knowing what else to do. The pain was slowly but irrevocably ratcheting up, and she was becoming desperate.

Description of pain is difficult because we do not have the vocabulary. Pain is therefore often described in similes. "It's like a knife stabbing" or "it's squeezing like a vice." Even the definition of pain is difficult to pin down. We all know what it is, but it's hard to put it into words.

There are two main types of physical pain: nociceptive and neuropathic. Nadia was experiencing both, but the latter would come to dominate her life for the next twenty years. There is also psychological pain—the subject for a story at another time.

Nociception is the normal sensation of a painful stimulus. It is a crucial function of the nervous system; without pain, we cannot learn to avoid damaging activities. Neuropathic pain is an abnormal sensation created by a damaged nervous system. The classic example would be "phantom limb pain" in an amputated limb.

Humans have evolved to have four different receptors in their skin and deep tissues that can detect touch, temperature, vibration and pain. Each of these sensations is transmitted from the skin to the brain through nerves. In the case of pain, the sensations travel through two different types of nerves. One is thick with insulation (myelin) and conducts sharp pain at high speeds; the second is thin, with no insulation, and conducts dull pain at much slower speeds. This is why, when you stub your toe, you feel an instantaneous sharp pain and then there is a short pause before the intense dull ache hits you in a second wave.

Without the pain system, it is difficult to survive. In the northern Swedish village of Vittangi, a number of people have been born with a congenital insensitivity to pain. Due to this genetic disorder, children can die from undetected infections, burns or injuries. Because they haven't experienced the negative consequence of pain, children do not fear jumping from high places and, if they reach adulthood, are often disabled from the broken bones accumulated from those mishaps.

Pain and learning are inextricably linked. We learn not to touch hot objects and typically remember that connection for the rest of our lives. Some societies have misguidedly used this association in their educational system, using corporal punishment to dissuade children from "bad behaviour." Those of us who endured schools with corporal punishment will remember the fear it provoked. Now the collateral damage of beating children in school—increased aggression, anti-social behaviour and mental health problems—has led to the practice being banned in most countries.

The association of pain and learning has some higher proponents. The Buddha is quoted as saying, "Pain is a gift; instead of avoiding it, learn to embrace it. Without pain, there is no growth."

Unfortunately, Nadia's pain was not teaching her any valuable lessons. When her husband returned, she swallowed two tablets of oxycodone. The powerful narcotic dissolved in her stomach and released its synthetic opioids into her bloodstream. Opioids are drugs that bind the opioid receptor and produce morphine-like effects. People have used morphine, found in the resin of the poppy plant, for millennia to treat pain or induce euphoria. Evidence of its use dates back to the Neolithic period. When the drug was first isolated from the opium poppy by Friedrich Sertürner in 1803, he named it after Morpheus, the Greek god of dreams and the son of Hypnos, the god of sleep, because of its tendency to induce slumber. Alongside its wonderful alleviation of pain, morphine and its more powerful modern synthetic cousins have numerous side effects, including respiratory depression. Overdose inhibits the sensation to breathe, and victims fall deeply asleep "in the arms of Morpheus," stop breathing (respiratory arrest) and die. The current opioid epidemic is a direct consequence of the drug's effects (euphoria) and side effects (respiratory arrest).

Nadia's pain was dulled slightly by the medications, but oxycodone nauseated her. The pain was throbbing deep in her right jaw, and it felt as if the bone was being squeezed in a vice and twisted. Any effort to bring relief was futile: She cried aloud but it did not help. She lay down because of the nausea, but the pain increased and pulsated up to the top of her head. She stood back up and almost fainted. Her vision greyed out and she buckled to one knee, and her husband leapt over to help her.

"We've got to take you to the emergency," he told her. He held her by the arm, and Nadia stumbled as they collected her things and made their way to the car.

In the emergency department, she waited several hours to be seen for several minutes. The emergency physician diagnosed post-operative pain and gave her a shot of fentanyl and Gravol. Fentanyl, an opioid one hundred times stronger than morphine, for the pain; Gravol for its expected nausea. Nadia fell asleep on the car ride home.

The next morning, she awoke to the horrible sensation that her jaw was on fire. It felt massively swollen; her tongue felt normal but the area of her chin and lower lip on the right side was still numb. Her tongue moved constantly searching for the source of pain. She took two oxycodone tablets before breakfast. The nausea distracted her hunger, and the pain was ramping up.

She phoned the endodontist's office and begged for an appointment, but the soonest he could see her was in several weeks. She phoned her dentist and was able to see him that afternoon.

In her dentist's office, she was in tears as she tried to describe the excruciating pain. The dentist listened, but his examination was strikingly normal. There was no more swelling than expected, and there was no obvious pus or signs of infection.

He diagnosed an infection and prescribed a course of antibiotics. Nadia returned home and endured another day of inconceivable pain.

A week later, she returned to the endodontist, who prescribed a second course of antibiotics. In reality, Nadia did not have an infection. She did not have a fever or redness or swelling at the site of the root canal. Her face felt swollen, but that was the result of nerve damage. In fact, considering her pain, her face looked remarkably normal in the mirror.

Two weeks later, she received a third course of antibiotics from her dentist. The diagnosis of infection was in part because he could not see how it could be anything else and in part because he needed to diagnose something. The antibiotics were, unfortunately, an unnecessary and useless exercise. Her pain was neuropathic.

Neuropathic pain was first recognized when people began to survive serious nerve injuries. In the American Civil War, surgeons learned to amputate mangled limbs with reproducible success, but amputees often complained of pain in their missing limb. The same phenomenon can plague transgender individuals in the most distressing way.

Doctors are just beginning to understand the neurophysiology underpinning neuropathic pain. If we truly understood it, we would predictably be able to correct it—and we can't. At least, that is the dogma written in every neurology textbook on pain. It is chronic and it is incurable. We can modify the pain, lessen it, but never completely alleviate it.

Why would a missing foot "hurt"? The following is an oversimplification of a very complex field, but it should elucidate the process. Pain gets from the foot to the brain through a relay of three nerves. Touch sensations also follow a parallel but different pathway. For pain, nerve number 1 goes from the foot to the spinal cord. It is straightforward and binary. The nerve either fires or it does not. Touch something painful, and it will fire a signal that reaches nerve number 2 in the spinal cord.

Nerve number 2 goes from the spinal cord to the thalamus (a relay station deep in the brain). Its firing is more complex and is modulated by several inputs. Most importantly, if nerve number 1 fires, nerve number 2 will fire and relay the message of pain towards the brain. Interestingly, touch sensations travelling in a nearby pathway send inhibitory signals to nerve number 2. Lots of touch sensations will therefore inhibit simultaneous pain sensation. This is why children rub their shin after accidentally banging it. They are flooding nerve number 2 with inhibition from touch sensation and thereby (partially) blocking the pain transmission. This is known as the gate control theory of pain. First described by Ronald Melzack and Patrick Wall in the 1960s, this theory postulates that only so much information can get through a gate in the spinal cord and reach the brain. This is likely the source of pain relief following touch and massage during child-birth. It is also the presumed mechanism of spinal cord stimulation—a new treatment for some lower-limb neuropathic pain.

Things can go terribly wrong with nerve number 2 if nerve number 1 dies (for example, following an amputation). First, when the parts of nerve number 1 touching nerve number 2 die off, the open spaces are filled in by other nearby nerves. That means a nerve carrying touch sensations may pathologically link up with nerve number 2. Now when that touch nerve is activated by brushing the skin with a gentle tissue, the information is processed up nerve number 2 and felt as pain. Light touch causing pain is called "allodynia," a characteristic of neuropathic pain.

Second, and more savage for the patient, when nerve number 2 stops receiving signals (from the dead nerve number 1), it begins to increase its ability to "hear" signals. It increases or upregulates the number and sensitivity of the receptors on its surface used for "listening." These new receptors can be so sensitive that they fire spontaneously and continuously. If nerve number 2 fires spontaneously, then the next nerve in the chain—nerve number 3—just relays the message to the brain. The sensation is felt as constant pain, even though nothing painful is touching the missing foot. A constant burning pain is another hallmark of neuropathic pain.

Nerve number 2 travels from the spinal cord up to the thalamus and contacts (at least) two different nerve 3s. Nerve 3a goes to the sensory cortex and tells us exactly where we felt the pain. We can localize the sensation to a pinprick or a stubbed toe. Nerve 3b goes to the limbic cortex and activates an emotional response to the pain. This is where we suffer from the pain. The potential dichotomy of pain and suffering has an anatomical substrate—they are felt in two different areas of the brain.

The Buddha's teachings are sometimes summarized, "Pain is inevitable. Suffering is optional." His teachings supported this dichotomy, and we are just starting to understand what that means. Without the limbic or emotional system, pain is just another sensation, like touch or temperature, without emotional context. You feel the sharp pain but do not care about it. Some older and more invasive neurosurgical procedures were designed to destroy the limbic pathways in patients with chronic pain. This burning-the-bridge approach was unfortunately caught in the appropriate backlash against lobotomy and fell out of favour. Control of the limbic system with Buddhist mindfulness can blunt pain in the same way anxiety or depression can magnify its perception.

This rudimentary understanding of the pathway for neuropathic pain can begin to suggest ways to ameliorate it. The key is to decrease or downregulate nerve number 2. Stop it from firing spontaneously and tricking nerve number 3 into thinking that there is constant pain.

More than a dozen anti-epileptic medications are used to stop seizures. They all work by reducing the ability of nerves to fire. These medications also help neuropathic pain. If it's felt somewhere on a scale of 1 to 10 (never 0), these medications turn the dial downwards. The unfortunate, ubiquitous side effect of these drugs is that they work indiscriminately on all nerve cells (neurons). Neurons in the frontal lobe, responsible for planning, are dulled. Neurons in the temporal lobe, responsible for memory, are dulled. Neurons in the brainstem, responsible for arousal or balance, are dulled. Patients report their pain level is reduced but at the expense of mental fogginess, poor memory and unsteady walking.

A year into Nadia's struggle, the pain had changed her. Once a talkative extrovert, she was now quiet and depressed. She had stopped working in a daycare centre because talking aggravated the pain, and she spent most of the day in a darkened room because bright lights worsened it too. She would not leave the house because the slightest wind on her face triggered severe pain (allodynia). Nothing made her happy; she was easily upset and chronically sad. At times she was suicidal, although she never formulated a plan to act on this impulse. She just wondered what the point of life was if she was just suffering.

Charles had seen the light in her eyes go out. Nadia was existing, not living.

She was taking an anti-epileptic medication and an antidepressant, but they both made her personality flat. She moved like a drunken zombie—slow, wobbly and stiff.

The pain was always there. She felt a constant, burning discomfort in her right lower teeth, lip and half her chin. The twisting pain in her lower jaw varied in intensity and could spread to include most of the right half of her face. At best, when the medications were strongest and she was her most stuporous, the pain was a 4. When the wind touched her face, the pain would ramp up to a 10. If she was quiet and alone, the pain would ease (but never go away); if she was anxious or upset, the pain escalated to excruciating. Many functions of the brain are ramped up by stress, including pain, depression and tremor—the latter is well known by any surgeon who has ever sensed a case was going poorly only to find their shaking hands making things even worse.

In 1990, eight years into her painful saga, her neurologist referred her to Dr. Peter Allen, an experienced neurosurgeon at the University of Alberta Hospital. At the time, he was the only neurosurgeon in Alberta using deep brain stimulation for pain. The popularity of DBS for pain would fade around the same time as its popularity for Parkinson's disease grew.

The concept was to block the pain in the thalamus, where nerve number 2 ended, and stop the signals reaching the higher parts of the brain where pain is felt. To achieve this, an insulated wire was inserted into the patient's thalamus and connected to a pacemaker in their chest. The pacemaker then provided an electrical current that travelled through the wire and was released through four small platinum contacts at its tip. The actual mechanism of pain relief was unknown, but the most popular suggestion at that time borrowed from the gate control theory—the idea that all the touch and pain sensations to the brain had to pass through a gate in the thalamus. The electricity from a DBS in the thalamus would flood the gate with touch signals and thereby reduce the amount of pain information that could get through. Patients reported a tingling sensation when the DBS was turned on, and this tingling sensation sometimes reduced the degree of pain they felt.

The popularity of DBS for pain rose rapidly in the early 1990s but quickly faded following two unsuccessful clinical trials. Initially there were lots of anecdotal case reports of its success, where patients reported benefit following DBS for a variety of painful conditions. But these successful reports lacked scientific credibility because they were not "blinded." In the excitement to get this new treatment licensed, the trials were poorly designed. Both the patient, and the person measuring the outcome (typically the surgeon), knew the patient had been treated. Under these circumstances, the placebo effect can have a powerful influence on the perceived outcome. The patient wants to get better and believes they will, and the surgeon wants the procedure to work. It may look like this:

"Are you sure you're still a 5 on the pain scale? You look much better than I have ever seen you. Are you not more of a 3?"

"Yes, Doctor. I feel more like a 3."

"Aha! I knew it would work."

The placebo effect is very real and powerful, especially in pain studies, where it can account for 30 percent of any result. It likely produces its effects through the body's natural pain-killing pathways. Morphine, a chemical from a plant, only works because it has a similar shape to a molecule that is found naturally in the body, namely, endogenous morphine, or endorphins, which provide pain relief during times of stress. There is a huge surge of endorphins during pregnancy, and their sudden post-partum reduction may play a role in post-partum depression—like a narcotic withdrawal.

The gold standard for a scientific study to prove a drug has an effect is now the randomized controlled trial, or RCT. First used to demonstrate that streptomycin could treat tuberculosis in 1948, the RCT removes the potential bias of the placebo effect. More importantly, the FDA will not license a drug without several positive RCTs. There are rare exceptions, such as the experimental drugs given during the Ebola outbreak in Liberia "on compassionate grounds" and the "emergency use authorization" of the vaccines for COVID-19.

To make the study blind, the RCT randomizes a group of test subjects into two arms: the experimental treatment group and the control group. Ideally there is no difference between these groups before the study begins. The experimental group receives the drug, and the control group receives a similar-looking placebo. Importantly neither group knows whether they have taken the drug or the placebo, thereby removing the placebo effect. Researchers measure the outcome at the end of the study, and the two groups are compared statistically to see if one did better.

Because of the poorly designed trials, the FDA refused to license DBS treatment for pain, insurance companies then refused to pay for the operation, and everyone stopped doing the procedure. The treatment died because of bad science, not necessarily because it didn't work.

Nadia met Dr. Allen during the hype that DBS could help neuropathic pain and a few years before the failed RCTs that suggested it could not. She does not remember much about the operation or about anything during those years, because she was drugged up with a mix of sedatives and a continuing cycle of different opioid painkillers.

After the operation, she had a pacemaker in her upper left chest and a new lump under her scalp at the top of the left side of her head. A hand-held controller allowed her to turn the device on when she woke up in the morning and off when she went to bed. When the DBS was on, she felt a tingling sensation in her right face, halfway between "pins and needles" and a buzzing sensation. When it was new, the sensation was quite strong, but it soon faded to a tolerable level and there were times, if she was really distracted, when she did not notice the tingling.

The first week after her surgery, the pain was better than it had ever been, and she was ecstatic. In hindsight this may have been due

to the lasting effect of the general anaesthetic given during the place-
ment of the pacemaker. The pain returned after a week, but it was still
better than she remembered, and she reported to Allen that the intensity had dropped to an average of 4/10.

Allen taught her how to adjust the "volume" of stimulation, which
changed the voltage output of the DBS. When her pain was particularly bad, she would click up a level or two. Emotionally, she liked this
option because it gave her some perceived control. She was no longer
a passive victim to the capricious whims of her pain. She had direct
access to it with her hand-held controller.

Again, in retrospect, this response may be difficult to tease apart
from placebo or a reduction in the suffering component of pain. The
same painful stimulus will be reported as being more painful if it is
associated with greater suffering due to depression and less painful if
the patient is happy.

Over the following year, Nadia slowly kept clicking up on her controller. Every month or so, she felt she needed more stimulation to get
the pain under control. By the end of the year, she had reached the
maximum setting.

The battery in a pacemaker lasts in an inverse proportion to the
output strength of its electrical current. For Nadia it was exhausted
after a year. She went to Alberta University Hospital to have a small
operation where the pacemaker in her chest was removed and replaced
with a new one. Dr. Allen set the DBS stimulation parameters, and
she was sent home the next day. This was not brain surgery; it was just
a pacemaker exchange.

Over the next year, she had her stimulation settings increased further, until her next pacemaker exchange ten months later. This cycle
continued for years, and then she moved with her husband to British
Columbia.

When I met Nadia, she'd had her thalamic DBS for more than ten years. My job was to replace the pacemaker when she needed a new one. To avoid confusion with the device that keeps the heart alive, these pacemakers were now called implantable neural stimulators, or INS. Our meetings were brief; she just needed a new INS every eight months because she was using such a high voltage it was consuming the battery quickly. I remember thinking she looked strikingly eccentric when I first met her. She wore large, dark glasses indoors with a scarf covering most of her face, like Jackie O avoiding the paparazzi. I later learned that light ramped up her pain and any breeze on her face burned like a flame.

Since I was the only neurosurgeon doing DBS operations in British Columbia, there was always a long waiting list of people who needed assessments, and it was not easy to get to see me. On several occasions Nadia's INS completely depleted and stopped working before I could replace it, and she realized that there was now no difference in her pain when the device was working or not. She didn't like the idea of giving up on this therapy but eventually was convinced it was not helping her. She asked me to remove the device.

I went over the various options. Leave it in place but turned off, remove the INS but leave the brain electrode in place, or remove everything and close that chapter in her life. She chose to have everything removed.

We discussed the risks of the procedure. DBS was still a relatively new treatment and I had not removed many electrodes from my patients; however, the few I had removed had all glided out of the brain easily with no complications. The electrodes were designed to be very smooth and were wrapped in silicone, except over the exposed platinum contacts. There were no rough edges for the brain to scar against, so removing them was simple.

I examined Nadia prior to her operation and found her generally healthy, with normal vital signs and a good heart and lungs. Her face was normal on the left side, but the right side was very abnormal. When I lightly touched her chin with a tissue, she reported it felt like sandpaper and glass raking her skin (allodynia). When I touched her with a pinprick, it felt like I was stabbing her with an icepick (hyperpathia). The area of abnormal sensation included her lower jaw and chin, but it had spread upwards in her cheek towards her eye and downwards into the upper part of her neck.

I expected the operation would be straightforward and planned to fit it in between two longer cases, since it would only take an hour at most. It turned out that the only difficult part was digging the wire out from under her scalp, as it had scarred into the tissues after being there for so long. The electrode in her brain gave the slightest suggestion of resistance, then pulled out smoothly. She was bundled off to the recovery room and I focused on the next case.

At the end of the day, I went to see her—and was horrified.

Nadia was lying in bed, mute and paralyzed on the right side of her body. I pinched her right hand, but it did not move. I asked her name, and she stared silently back at me. She was spontaneously moving her left arm and leg, but nothing on the right side.

I assumed she had suffered a thalamic hemorrhage from the operation, and organized a stat CT scan of her head. We raced her down to the CT scanner in her hospital bed. The nurse was apologizing for not calling us earlier, but I didn't say anything. I was deeply concerned about the potentially devastating consequence of a hemorrhage.

The left thalamus is situated close to the main pathway from the left motor cortex that controls the right side of the body; her paralyzed state suggested the hemorrhage must have been big. The left thalamus also has many connections with the language and cognitive centres of the brain. Nadia would not be able to talk—worse, she might not be able to think.

We transferred her to the CT gantry, and the technician lined up her head with a red laser light while I waited in the control booth for the images to come out.

They started to appear on the computer screen one slice at a time, starting with the bottom of the head and working upwards. The first scan, far below where I had pulled out the electrode, looked normal (as expected). I winced and gritted my teeth as the slices got closer to the thalamus.

The bottom thalamic slice appeared on the screen and nothing was abnormal—just various shades of grey. The next two slices were also normal. The one after that had a tiny white dot where the electrode would have been. The white dot was blood—a hemorrhage. The next slice after that had a four-millimetre white dot in the tract where I had pulled out the electrode. The rest were normal.

There was a hemorrhage right where the tip of the electrode had been, but it was tiny. This was immediately reassuring but also confusing. It was tiny and I could reassure her (if she could understand me) that she should get better. How much better, I did not know. I was surprised she had such a profound deficit from such a small stroke. It didn't make sense, but in truth, I had not seen a lot of thalamic strokes.

We wheeled her back up to the recovery room, and I went to talk to her husband, feeling some dread. It is painful to begin a conversation with, "Your wife has had a stroke during my operation . . ."

I found him in the waiting room and sat beside him. He lowered his newspaper and I began, "We got all the hardware out fine, but there is a very small hemorrhage at the site of the electrode."

"What does that mean?"

"There is a very small amount of bleeding where the electrode used to be. It has stopped, but her brain does not like it."

"Okay?" he asked.

"She is going to get better, but first she will get worse. Do you understand?"

"Yes," he responded, but he really didn't.

"The brain does not like any bleeding and it will swell in response. When you bang your knee, it is always worse the next day before it gets better."

"Will she get better?"

"Of course." I was reassuring him more than I should. "But we will have to wait and see if she completely recovers." When I introduced the concept that she could be permanently injured, he began to grasp the situation.

"How bad is she?"

"Right now, she is pretty bad. She can't move her right side and she can't talk." I dropped the bombshell.

"What?"

"The electrode has caused some bleeding when it came out," I began again, subconsciously blaming the electrode rather than me. "Right now, Nadia isn't talking or moving much."

"Oh my God." He was starting to understand.

"I've scanned her already and the bleeding is very small."

"You've scanned her?"

"Yes."

"And the bleeding is small?"

"Yes."

"What does that mean?"

"Nadia has had a small bleed and she will need some time to recover."

"Okay. What does that mean?"

"It means she needs some rest tonight and then we will scan her again in the morning."

"Okay. Will she be okay?"

"Yes. We will look after her and check her again in the morning."
I sat right beside him and leaned in as I spoke. Lots of head nodding.

"Thanks, Doc."

"No worries. We'll look after her." I shook his hand with both
of mine.

My primary concerns at that time were with Nadia, not her husband. Why had she bled? What did I do wrong?

I would learn the answer that evening. The INS had a lithium battery in it, so it was sent back to the manufacturer to be discarded
environmentally, but the OR nurses weren't sure what to do with the
brain electrode. It was made of platinum, and they wanted to know if
it should be recycled or thrown out. I went back up to the OR to sort
this out, and when I looked at it closely, it was slightly different from
any of the electrodes I had used for my DBS cases. It turned out to be
a first-generation electrode, and protruding from its tip was a small
loop of wire, which engineers called contact o because it looked like a
zero. The second generation of electrodes, the only ones I had ever
seen, no longer had this two-millimetre-diameter loop. All the contacts (four per electrode) were smooth cylinders of platinum with no
edges or loops for the brain to scar against. When I pulled out Nadia's
electrode, the tiny scar of tissue that had grown through the loop was
torn away and started some bleeding.

I now understood the how and why, but I still couldn't make sense
of what was happening to Nadia. The discrepancy between her profound deficit and the small hemorrhage on her CT scan tormented me
that night. I dreamt about the operation all night and awoke several
times at the moment of the pull.

The next morning, I headed in to work and went straight to her
bedside.

She was sitting up in bed with a half-eaten tray of breakfast in front of her. She smiled when I came in and her smile was almost symmetrical (no right facial weakness). She was holding a spoon in her right hand!

I was stunned. She was not paralyzed—she was moving her right side!

I lifted up my arms and wiggled my fingers and she mimicked me. I asked her to show me how she used her spoon and she scooped some red Jell-O into her spoon and ate it.

"That's great!" I was elated. "Can you speak?"

She shook her head from side to side as a no. She clearly understood me but was unable to formulate any words, though she was smiling. Her inability to speak didn't make sense to me at the time, but I was happy that she was happy.

My conversation with her husband was easier. "She is moving her arm much better now and it's been less than a day."

"Is that good, Doc?"

"Yes. That's very good. Better than expected. We'll have to wait to see about her speech. It might be slurred when it comes back."

"When will it come back?"

"I don't know."

"When will we be able to go home?" The inappropriateness of the question surprised me. He did not have a clear grasp of the severity of Nadia's situation. I knew I had been overly optimistic, but he was not getting it. Twelve hours ago, Nadia was looking at a long-term care home. Now she might need a few months of rehab before she went home.

I was distracted with a number of other patients and did not return to see Nadia until the next afternoon. When I got to her room, she was sitting in a chair talking to her husband. Talking!

I sat on the edge of the bed looking at her. "How are you doing?"

"Great!" She was beaming. Her whole face was smiling.

"Great?" I was completely perplexed. Why was she so happy after a near-fatal complication? Perhaps it was just the relief of knowing she would not be paralyzed. "How is the coordination in your hand?"

She did not answer my question. Instead she bowed her head and leant forwards. She was smirking and looked like she wanted to tell me something. It made me instantly nervous—what could be wrong now? She clasped her hands between her knees, looked up at me and said, "I am pain-free."

I asked what she meant.

"For the first time in twenty years, my face is pain-free." She was slow and deliberate with her words.

"What do you mean 'pain-free'?"

"I mean, I have absolutely no pain in my face." She could not have been clearer.

"I have never heard of that," I finally said. "It's . . . it's . . ."

"It's a miracle!" she finished my sentence.

Nadia left hospital a few days later. I expected to get a call from her telling me the pain was back, but I never did. Five years later, I decided to investigate the exact location of her brain hemorrhage because it must have been the source of (or pathway from) her chronic neuropathic pain. Perhaps we could deliberately destroy or modulate that part of the brain in other patients with the same type of pain. In 2021, we submitted a medical paper using a new DBS that could steer the current precisely into "Nadia's target" and had dramatically reduced the neuropathic dental pain in another patient. Following this proof-of-concept report, we are now undertaking a study with our Swiss colleagues to see if this technique can reduce dental neuropathic pain in a larger group of patients suffering from this condition.

The total resolution of neuropathic pain following a dental injury is unheard of. It can be reduced. It can be less associated with suffering.

It can be tolerated. But I have never seen a patient or read a report of it being completely alleviated. For me this was a miracle. A surprising and welcomed event that cannot be explained by natural or scientific laws and is therefore considered to be the work of a divine agency.

A "welcomed event" is of course a gross understatement, because I thought I had disabled her for life. Thalamic strokes are notoriously disabling (particularly on the dominant left side). Nadia's hemorrhage destroyed her dental pain centre, and the resultant temporary swelling around the hemorrhage pushed on and blocked the nearby functions of her body's movement and speech. When the swelling settled and the pressure on nearby structures relaxed, her movement and speech returned. No wonder thalamic strokes can be catastrophic: these crucial nearby structures are very close together, only the distance of some swelling apart.

In the next decade, when we are more knowledgeable about the thalamic pain centre, Nadia's miraculous result might be expected. I sometimes wonder, however, if her journey might have been guided by a divine providence, although that is hard to reconcile with my scientific background. We have more accurate imaging and targeting systems than ever before, and clearly a few millimetres matters. Now we can place an electrode in the brain within two millimetres. This new accuracy and Nadia's small target area may open a new field of neurosurgery designed to reliably alleviate dental neuropathic pain.

Her transformation from paralyzed and mute to pain-free and independent was as stunning as it was inexplicable. I could not explain it, but it happened. Since it happened, and now that we're studying the outcome, I hope one day it can be explained. Nadia's miracle may be a future patient's salvation.

Meanwhile, Nadia's miracle has humbled me. There is so much we do not know about the brain that is waiting to be discovered. The study of neurosurgery has allowed me to glimpse new truths about brain function; the practice of neurosurgery has allowed me to see new truths about myself. The final story, about Alan and his brain tumour, taught me more about myself than him.

12.

ALAN & ME

In 1792, Dionisio Alcalá-Galiano sailed by the island on the west coast of British Columbia that now bears his name while commanding the schooner *Sutil* as part of Spain's mission to find a Northwest Passage around North America. In June of that year, he met the British naval officer Captain George Vancouver, who was on a similar mission aboard HMS *Discovery*. Two men from different worlds but with a common purpose.

Remarkably they got along and shared their maps, despite the animosity between Spain and England. Vancouver would die in obscurity only six years later, embroiled in a legal battle with the cousin of the British prime minister, whom he had disciplined and ultimately dismissed from the voyage. Galiano would die a few years later off the coast of Spain in the great naval battle of Trafalgar.

These days, Galiano Island has approximately one thousand residents, many of whom are passionate environmentalists or descendants of the 1960s counterculture movement. In January 2001, a rock band from Vancouver played at the island's town hall to honour one of the residents. Shortly thereafter, the rhythm guitarist would be diagnosed with a brain tumour. This is the story of how he radically changed my perspective on medicine.

Alan's medical drama began on a half-frozen soccer field in mid-February 2001, when he was forty-nine years old. On the west coast of Canada, the mild climate allows soccer to be played year-round, and as a result, the quality of play is surprisingly good. During the game, Alan went up for a header, got bumped and fell backwards, hitting the back of his head—a particularly dangerous way to hit your head because it can damage the spinal cord. The rabbit punch, a deliberate blow to the back of the head, was banned in boxing by the Marquess of Queensberry in 1867 for this very reason. The referee of an amateur soccer game in Detroit in 2014 was killed by a disgruntled player with just such a punch.

Alan thought he might have blacked out for an instant, but he got up and kept playing. He was the central defender, after all, the last line of defence, and he would never lie down or quit. Ever since breaking both wrists after jumping off a garage roof at age six, he'd accepted that injuries accompanied adventurous behaviour. He was the team captain type, a strong competitor who had grown up playing against his older brother's friends. To prove you were tough, you prevailed in silence.

A few months later, on April 16—on the morning after another soccer match—he woke strangely early, around 5 a.m., and knew something was odd. He was unable to move his right index finger, and his balance was slightly off. He felt disoriented, not fully himself, and tiptoed downstairs trying not to disturb his wife. They lived on a quiet street in Vancouver's westside. It was now spring; the birds were singing and there were delicate white blossoms on their pear tree. In his bare feet, wearing a white dressing gown, he walked across the wet grass into the garage he had converted into a backyard office.

At this stage of his life, as a self-employed writer, he was someone who had to work every day. Eventually he would go on to publish twenty books and receive Canada's highest civilian honour, the Order of Canada, for his work, but in 2001 he was still struggling to make ends meet. He did not understand what was wrong with him that morning, so he tried to distract himself with work. Denying weakness or injury had always worked in the past.

When Alan sat down at his desk, he realized he couldn't easily move the individual fingers of his right hand to type. He kept trying but they would not co-operate. Finally he admitted to himself that something was seriously amiss but remained determined not to make a fuss about it. The younger of his two sons had a bedroom in the basement, and he walked back across the yard and into the house, intending to alert his son.

Alan stood at the top of the stairs leading down to the basement and paused, ready to call out, but realized he could not remember his son's name. He held onto the door frame, bowed his head, and tried to remember the name of his older son, the one who was in Japan. He could not remember his name either.

Something was very, very wrong. He needed his wife. Alan made it back upstairs. His garbled words and wide eyes spoke volumes. Tara was awake in an instant and took charge. They had married in their early twenties, and it was a great comfort knowing his wife was an extremely sensible and competent person, the boss of their domesticity.

They lived about a ten-minute drive from Vancouver General, and Tara drove him there with little conversation. Halfway to the hospital, as his ability to speak began to return, Alan told Tara what had happened the day before at the soccer game in Richmond. The opposing goalkeeper had a booming kick that could reach beyond the midfield, and after one particularly dizzying launch, Alan had the temerity to head the ball back towards the opponents' half. He wondered if he might have somehow "dislodged" something when he headed that ball or perhaps when he fell on that frozen pitch a few months ago.

By the time they parked and walked into the emergency department at 6:30 a.m., Alan's ability to speak had fully returned to normal. He could have shrugged off the mysterious symptoms and pretended all was now fine, but he knew better. He would let Tara do the talking. The triage nurse met them and wrote "possible concussion" on his chart. Alan underwent a battery of tests over the next several hours. Most vital was his CT scan around noon.

—⬛—

As the neurosurgeon on call that day, I was introduced to Alan's brain before I met him. His CT was routinely reviewed by a radiologist, and the final line of her report concluded with the message ". . . call neurosurgery." My pager went off, and I was summoned from the OR to the darkened cavern of the radiology reporting room, always dimly lit to facilitate seeing the radiology images.

There were six desks with a small crowd of medics huddling around each one, their faces buried in a forest of illuminated monitors. From behind, where I stood when I came in, the tops and sides of their hair were lit blue from the screens. I waited for my eyes to adapt to the dark.

The light from the door opening signalled my arrival, and they called me over. I sat beside the radiologist in the middle of the cohort and reviewed Alan's brain scan. There was a five-centimetre spherical extra-axial mass compressing the left motor cortex. The tumour was the size of a small orange and roughly the same shape. It was inside the skull but outside the brain—hence extra-axial. I knew the most common tumour in this location was a meningioma, a tumour of the meninges that covered the brain, as we saw with Mr. Ouamouno in Liberia. First named by Cushing, it was most often benign.

As these tumours grow, they push against the skull, which does not move, and against the brain, which does. Their slow growth allows the brain to get out of the way. But eventually the brain cannot tolerate any further compression and it objects with headaches, seizures or strokes. We reviewed the tumour's blood supply and how it was compressing the left motor cortex, the part of the brain Penfield had elegantly shown was responsible for movement of the right side of the body.

As I got up to leave, one of the young medical students eagerly asked, "What are you going to do?"

"Take it out."

Definitive. Curative. As with the thoracic surgeon who'd fixed Jeff all those years ago, the answer was as simple as the procedure was complex.

"But what about the motor cortex?" In a hurry to get back to the operating room, I left without answering.

After I finished my second operation of the day, I walked down to the emergency department to meet the brain tumour. As I mentioned at the outset, science should prevail over sentiment in medicine, for the sake of the patient. I therefore knew what I was going to say, based on analysis and reason, before I encountered the person in whom the brain tumour was embedded. Normally that was a good thing.

I had decided in advance that I would not divulge the full details of what I knew. I did not want to scare the patient away from choosing the right course. My job was to reassure him that I could help him, that I knew the pathway he should take, and to send him on his way to await surgery. I had allotted about ten minutes.

When I met Alan, I had absolutely no idea that after more than a thousand operations, he would be the first patient with whom I would let my clinical guard down and become close friends. The conversation began more or less as planned. I told him what the ER physician had already told him: he had a brain tumour, a pretty big one, on the left, near the part that controlled the right-hand side and his speech. I added that I suspected the tumour was a meningioma and that it was *probably* benign. We would have more information after his MRI, but ultimately, we would need a piece of the growth to know exactly what it was.

Tara explained that Alan was not a reliable barometer when it came to reporting any frailties or mishaps. He was no stranger to emergency wards, but if you asked him for a list of ailments, he genuinely wouldn't recall half of them. I appreciated her candour—it made my job easier when I had all the facts.

I explained that his symptoms this morning had likely been a seizure, not a stroke. The bizarre forgetfulness, temporary speech loss and weakness of the right hand had all resolved, but could happen again. He should therefore be taking Dilantin, one of the most common and effective anti-seizure medications. To further encourage their acquiescence and optimism, I ventured that his situation was so straightforward that we could even remove the tumour immediately, if he wanted.

I was taken aback by Alan's response.

"Okay, let's do it."

He was fully prepared to get it over with, on the spot, no dilly-dallying. I had never come across this before. His eagerness was genuine: he had sized me up, while his wife and I were talking, and he trusted me. He was far less interested in getting a medical diagnosis and an anatomy lesson than he was in evaluating me—as if our roles had been reversed and I was the one who was really under scrutiny. Evidently he liked what he saw and felt there was no point in delaying the inevitable. Game on.

I had to backtrack.

Fortunately Tara was equally opposed to any hasty approach. I explained that in Alan's case it would be prudent (translation: necessary) to employ a technique called cortical mapping, which would entail additional personnel and expertise. As I tried to vaguely explain cortical mapping, an astute patient could ascertain that a good deal of danger was being assessed. If additional personnel would be required to conduct an independent monitoring of his brain while I was operating—*Hey, Chris, whatever you do, don't cut there!*—well, the tumour was not as easy to remove as I had first suggested. The size and location of his tumour *were* problematic.

That evening, while his wife went to pick up the prescription for his anti-seizure medication, Alan had the most excruciating headache he had ever had. His swollen brain was pushing out against his dura. The brain does not have pain sensors, but the dura surrounding it has lots (as everyone with migraines knows only too well). By the next day, he was pain-free and able to function again—the calm before the storm.

A date for surgery was set. Alan and Tara took a respite on a communally owned, wooded property on Galiano. I did not give his case much more thought. We had one additional meeting in my office before the surgery, and Alan seemed philosophical about his situation, perhaps unusually objective. He articulated that one of the most bizarre moments of his life—forgetting the names of his sons—may have been a godsend. Playing soccer had resulted in an early warning about the presence of the previously asymptomatic tumour. Far from being disconsolate, he considered himself fortunate. He said he had the love of his family and about three or four lifetimes of experience and adventures, and he was grateful to have had such bounty. He had, to put it mildly, a very positive attitude.

I confess I was not at all interested in these philosophical conjectures. I was accustomed to being the professor during these conversations;

I did not want to be taught by a patient. Whether or not he was afraid of death really didn't have much to do with my job. Tara, sensing a growing tension between us in the same small room, tried to ameliorate the situation and steer us towards neutral ground.

To defray Alan's philosophical tangents, I reassured the couple this would be a meat-and-potatoes operation. Alan seemed to take offence at any inference that his surgery might be ordinary. If it really was a simple procedure, why hadn't I proceeded when we first met, as I had suggested? He was right. There was no animosity on his part. On the contrary, I could sense he liked and respected me; he was not in the least averse to having me as his brain surgeon. He was glad it was me. He just refused to be the subservient party.

———

The next time I met Alan was the day of his surgery, May 28. Just prior to his brain surgery, when he was being prepared in a hospital gown, he was happily reading the *New York Review of Books*.

For his operation I would follow the same philosophy as when I performed the brain tumour removal on Mr. Ouamouno in Liberia thirteen years later. There were two differences. First, the location of Alan's tumour—directly over and compressing his motor cortex—was more dangerous. Any damage to that part of the brain would leave him paralyzed on his right side. Second, the equipment to visualize and remove Alan's tumour was far better. The first factor was not in my favour. The second was.

The operation took five hours. There was an alternating dance of aggressive force and subtle touch during this surgery. I drilled a window through the hard bone of his skull with a high-speed drill to reveal the soft structures beneath. The tumour itself was as firm as a stone. It had pushed the soft brain away over many years of growth, until the brain could take no further distortion and had protested in a storm of electrical activity. I removed the bulk of the tumour quickly, coring out its centre, which was the farthest away from the delicate brain and could be removed aggressively. But the edge of the tumour, where it pressed into Alan's motor cortex, had to be peeled away from his brain very, very slowly. That crucial interface, where the tumour met his brain, was where mistakes would cause paralysis.

I felt the removal of the tumour was a personal battle between the cancer and myself. There was success or failure—I had not yet met and learned from Saika. At the time I was treating Alan, I expected to win but knew that sometimes it was impossible. Sun Tzu, the Chinese military leader in the fifth century BCE, wrote, "It is said that if you know your enemies and know yourself, you will not be imperilled in a hundred battles." The operating microscope and cortical mapping allowed me to know my enemies.

The tumour had many tricks, but at high magnification under the microscope, it was hard to hide them. The boundary between the tumour and brain should be obvious, but when the brain is squeezed so hard that it looks abnormal, then the boundary becomes unclear. Straying during the dissection into the abnormal-looking brain would cause strokes. I knew what an abnormal brain looked like and proceeded with caution.

The vessels feeding the tumour (which needed to be coagulated and cut) would occasionally also feed the brain. These en passant vessels were a deadly trap, and sacrificing them caused strokes. The first time you learn this rule is shocking: your patient wakes up paralyzed. As your battle experience grows, the distinction between arteries that feed the brain or the tumour, or that feed both, becomes obvious. As your confidence grows and you begin to relax, the tumours have one last trick—the veins.

By the time I met Alan, I had already learned (the hard way) that sacrificing a vein can be catastrophic. Today I would sacrifice no vessel unless forced. This prolonged the case, because it was technically challenging to protect vulnerable vessels while carving out a rock-hard tumour. The tumour was beaten slowly on multiple fronts. I had to advance where it was easy and then stop. Redirect to another front and progress there until it became too difficult. It was my choice where and when to attack; the tumour had to wait and hide its defences.

Eventually it was all out. Alan's head was put back together, and he was bundled off to the neurosurgical intensive care unit. A few hours later, Alan asked the attending nurse for a pencil and paper. He needed to write down what was happening.

In another bed, a recovering patient across from him was attempting to climb out of her bed after her surgery. The nurse in charge told Alan that this patient was an avid mountaineer. People recovering from serious operations under heavy medication frequently instinctually resort to behaviour at which they excelled. Alan tried to pick up the pencil.

He could not yet use his right hand—it simply didn't work. Unperturbed, he etched out the words with his left hand. These were messages for the various people he loved, printed with his left hand, in the dark, between midnight and 4 a.m. These scribblings were reproduced, like cave drawings, in the memoir that he would later publish, a thin book called *Intensive Care*—an affirmation of how the imminence of death can greatly enhance life.

A few days after the operation, I went to see Alan as he was recovering in Room 525. Instead of pajamas, he was wearing a red-and-white-striped Tolteca Guadalajara soccer jersey that a friend had bought for him in Mexico. He was now completely bald, with a major gash on his scalp, but he was entirely upbeat, talking fast because he said he didn't want to waste too much of my time. Taped to the door was a photo of the bald French goalkeeper, Barthez, who had won the World Cup with Zidane. Pleased with the result of the surgery, I wished him well and presumed we wouldn't meet again. I don't remember having any significant conversation. We stood side by side under the fluorescent lights of the cold ward, surrounded by nurses, and paused for a picture.

About a year later, Alan sent me a copy of *Intensive Care*. I read it knowing I had won the battle against his tumour. My victory was anatomical; his was a renewed quality of life. At that point in my career, I felt my successes were all under the microscope. In this case the tumour had conceded I was better. I had made no mistakes. Flawless. I had not yet learned to translate these microscopic battles into the macroscopic world where someone's life was better at the end of the day.

But it turned out there was more to the story than that operation.

Alan's seizures began soon after he got back home. His brain was moving back to its original position, and it was protesting the distortions. At first the seizures were confined to his hand—what doctors call a focal motor seizure. The small muscles of his hand would twitch rhythmically and then pull hard into a fist, and there was nothing at all he could do about it. After a minute it passed, leaving his hand a bit weak and sore for an hour.

The first grand mal seizure—what doctors call a focal seizure with secondary generalization—happened on a Saturday afternoon. It began in his right hand—they always did—and his fingers curled into a useless claw. Then his wrist and arm flexed into a body builder's posture. He could feel an uncomfortable tightness flowing up his arm like an unstoppable wave rolling across the ocean. As the electrical storm spread across his motor cortex, the next part of his body contracted fully. The seizure marched up his right arm like Hannibal's elephants marching up and over the Alps. He tried to grab onto something with his left hand, but the squeezing pressure flowed over his right shoulder and onto his torso. He was shaking and the right side of his face begin to tighten, at first rhythmically and then just pulling. He tried to cry out, but he knew it was already too late. The wave attacked his mouth and the seizure robbed him of speech. The electrical storm in his brain then spread across his corpus callosum to the other side and he lost consciousness.

This first grand mal seizure was particularly traumatizing. Alan and his wife had not been warned what it might be like or even that it might happen. Tara managed to somehow get Alan into the back seat of a car while their friend Dale, who happened to be visiting, called 911. It was midday, but it felt like a nightmare. The dispatcher at 911 advised them to pull over and wait for the ambulance. Parked at the intersection of Macdonald and West 12th Avenue, halfway between their home and the hospital, Tara worried that her husband was dying. Why was the ambulance taking so long? They could be there already if they hadn't stopped.

They arrived back at Vancouver General during a labour dispute. The overworked nurses had been without a contract for months, and there were more patients on gurneys in the corridors than usual. Alan's seizure had stopped and he would just have to wait. He was one of many.

On a stretcher next to him was a self-described alcoholic who had been mugged. She was an experienced sufferer. Alan felt an unforeseen kinship. This woman knew to remain calm. She had reached a stage in her gentle and sad life where she could comfortably blame every misfortune on herself. They talked, and she told Alan she would pray for him. When she suddenly stopped talking and closed her eyes, Alan managed to point out to the staff that his fellow patient had lost consciousness.

Alan had another seizure, and by the time they brought him Ativan, the drug used to stop seizures rapidly, he was shaking too violently to get it under his tongue. He lay on his side, shaking the gurney, staring at the stomach of a large ambulance attendant in a white shirt. This was very different from the small hand-twitching that occurred in private. This seizure was happening in public, alongside the destitute alcoholic and just down the hallway from Parmish, a South Asian schizophrenic surrounded by two grim policemen.

Alan's entire body was now in a sustained contraction. He was not breathing normally; every rib and abdominal muscle contracted in a prolonged exhalation. His body began to jerk rhythmically; he had felt the wave coming all the time, but only now was it crashing on the shore for everyone else to notice. This sensation of helpless loneliness within the cyclone of the grand mal seizure was far more alarming to him than the prospect of brain surgery had been.

His body felt as if it was being transformed into an out-of-control racing car, and he feared he would do permanent damage as he watched the RPM needle on the dash rising and rising. But then the seizure spontaneously stopped, and Alan's senses gradually returned. The first thing he realized was that all his muscles hurt and he had a bad headache. He blinked and tried to focus his eyes. He tried to lift his head up and speak but could only manage a mumble. He knew what he wanted to say but could not coordinate his mouth to say it. Eventually his speech returned, and he was sent upstairs to recover.

The next day a nurse removed the surgical staples from his head. He told her he was glad he had had the big seizure, because now he knew what it was like for people with epilepsy. "A seizure," he told her, "is like an enema for your pride." Eventually, Alan would devote four years to writing a biography about a female doctor who had worked with Albert Schweitzer and pioneered the successful treatment of epilepsy, in a rural area of Tanzania where the incidence of the condition was ten times higher than the global norm.

—

Seizures were originally associated with the gods, or supernatural powers. At the time of Hippocrates a volume was written called *On the Sacred Disease.* The author is unknown, but it's possible that it was written by the father of medicine himself. In it, the author dismissed the prevailing view that the disease was a punishment from the gods and put forth the theory that it was due to a very human ailment of having too much phlegm choking the brain.

We may mock this phlegm theory, just as the author mocked the sacred theory, but it was a momentous moment in medicine. For a thousand years before Hippocrates, beginning with the Babylonians, the cause of seizures was unknown and therefore ascribed to the supernatural. The Babylonians recognized several different types of seizures and felt each was due to a specific evil spirit. Their laws, the first ever to be written down (by Hammurabi in 1750 BCE), prohibited people with seizures from marrying or voting. The understanding of seizures was a template for the (lack of) understanding of most aspects of medicine—we don't understand it, therefore it must be controlled by the gods. Hippocrates or the book's unknown author shattered this supernatural concept in the book. Of seizures, it says:

> Men regard its nature and cause as divine from ignorance
> and wonder because it is not at all like other diseases. . . .
> Neither truly do I count it a worthy opinion to hold that the
> body of man is polluted by god, the most impure by the
> most holy.

It was revolutionary at the time to believe that this illness had a physical cause. The author turned out to be wrong about that physical cause—a blockage of phlegm leaving the brain through its veins—but this theory fit the knowledge of the time and did explain some of the well-known aspects of seizures. For example, children often died of their seizures, whereas older people typically did not; the author theorized that the veins of children were smaller and therefore clogged with phlegm more easily. We now know the most common seizure in infants is from hypoxia (lack of oxygen) at birth, which is often a lethal event. The most common seizure in older people follows a small stroke, which is often survivable.

The author confirmed that the source of the seizure was the brain, continuing:

> Men ought to know that from nothing else but the brain
> come joys, delights, laughter and sports, and sorrows, griefs,
> despondency, and lamentations. And by this, in an especial
> manner, we acquire wisdom and knowledge, and see and
> hear, and know what are foul and what are fair, what are
> bad and what are good.

This approach removed some of the stigma associated with seizures and the disease of repeated seizures, which was called epilepsy (from the Greek "to take hold of" or "to seize"). Unfortunately, humankind would undo much of this good work over the next thousand years. It would often be presumed that if epilepsy was a sacred disease, and therefore given to someone because the gods felt they deserved it, then that person must be evil. This view is apparent in the Bible, and it spread through the Middle Ages as the Bible became a reference for all aspects of life in Europe.

In the Gospel of Mark 9:17–18, Jesus met a boy possessed with an evil spirit. The boy's father describes his symptoms, which are now familiar to us as epilepsy.

> A man in the crowd answered, "Teacher, I brought you my son, who is possessed by a spirit that has robbed him of speech. Whenever it seizes him, it throws him to the ground. He foams at the mouth, gnashes his teeth and becomes rigid. I asked your disciples to drive out the spirit, but they could not."

Jesus rebuked the spirit and commanded it to leave the boy and never return. The boy recovered from his seizure and was able to get up. Unfortunately, we are not given any long-term follow-up for this case report.

The Gospel of Mark (written anonymously around 70 CE) was the first of the four canonical gospels, followed by Matthew and Luke (who copied many of the stories of Jesus) and later John. The story of the boy with epilepsy appears in both Matthew 17:14–21 and Luke 9:37–45. The version in the Gospel of Matthew adds that the boy was "moonstruck," a reference to the concept that diseases that repeated at intervals were thought to be influenced by the moon. The King James Version of the New Testament would translate the term as "lunatick," from the Latin word *lunaticus*. Our word "lunatic," of unsound mind, derives from this origin and has permeated literature and the law ever since. The word was only removed from all laws in the United States under President Obama in 2012.

The Bible's interpretation of the cause of epilepsy guided the public's understanding throughout the Middle Ages. If epilepsy was caused by an evil spirit, then perhaps appealing to a saint could cure it. Consequently, St. Valentine—named for Valentinus, a physician and priest in early Rome—is the patron saint for those seeking relief from both loneliness and epilepsy. There may have been several Valentines over the years who have become incorporated into the story of one person. Valentinus refused to renounce Christianity and was beheaded on the day that still bears his name, February 14, 270 CE. Why Valentinus became associated with epilepsy may relate to the similar sound of his name and the German word for "fallen." He was not the patron saint of epilepsy in medieval France (where it was St. John) or England (where it was St. Paul), but he was in Germany.

Our current understanding of epilepsy did not begin until the nineteenth century. In 1873 the English neurologist John Hughlings Jackson (one of the three neurologists who watched Macewen remove the first intracranial tumour) published his *Study of Convulsions*. In it, he wrote, "Epilepsy is the name for occasional, sudden, excessive, rapid and local discharges of grey matter." Jackson described the march of a focal seizure through the body and correctly suggested that the brain must therefore have discrete areas responsible for movement of a body part and that these areas must be connected (later proven by Penfield during awake brain surgery). An epileptic storm ranging through the brain sequentially activates these areas, causing the spread of body contractions that Alan had suffered in the emergency department. That spread of a seizure from the thumb to the hand to the arm to the body would become known as a "Jacksonian seizure."

Jackson married his cousin, Elizabeth. Unfortunately, in a cruel twist of fate, she developed Jacksonian seizures three years after her husband first described them and shortly before she died of a cerebral venous thrombosis.

Knowledge of epilepsy exploded around that time. Gustav Theodor Fritsch and Eduard Hitzig showed that seizures could be triggered in dogs by electrical stimulation of their brains. Hippocrates—if it was he—had been correct in assuming the brain was the site of seizures, and now physicians knew electricity was its source.

The German psychiatrist Hans Berger introduced the *Elektrenkephalogramm*, or EEG, which could record the electrical activity of the brain in order to recognize and classify seizures. Berger was obsessed with the ability of the brain to transmit its thoughts by telepathy. He had fallen from his horse in a cavalry training exercise and a horse-drawn cannon had stopped inches from killing him. That day his sister, miles away, sensed something terrible had happened to him and convinced their father to send him a telegram.

The event left a lasting impression on the young Berger, who decided to study medicine with the goal of understanding psychic energy. He used silver wires to detect the electrical activity of the brain in a patient who had a hole trepanned in his skull prior to surgery. The very small amplitude of the brain's electrical activity (measured in thousands of a volt) is usually obscured by the thick skull. In this case, he was able to record it with the EEG and see it change with different brain activity. The discovery would eventually revolutionize the fields of epilepsy and sleep science. Berger, however, would have a sad life, culminating in suicide by hanging at age sixty-eight.

The first successful medication for seizures was potassium bromide, which was found, like most discoveries in medicine, by chance. Some seizures were felt at the time to be due to sexual excitement, and potassium bromide caused impotence—a less severe preventative treatment than castration, which was also used. Unbeknownst to the physicians who prescribed it, potassium bromide also inhibited neurons from electrically firing, thereby reducing the likelihood of spreading a seizure. Therefore, potassium bromide became the drug of choice for epilepsy from 1857 to the discovery of phenobarbital in 1912. It is still used for epilepsy in dogs.

A young German psychiatrist, Alfred Hauptmann, used phenobarbital, which was originally marketed by Bayer as a sedative, to sedate some epileptics, and it unexpectedly reduced their seizures. It became the drug of choice for epilepsy for the next fifty years. Dilantin (phenytoin) was approved by the FDA in 1958 and continues to be a standard medication for generalized seizures.

———

"All of me, why not take all of me . . ."

After Alan's grand mal seizure, he went home and stayed in bed for at least a month, frequently listening over and over to a tape of Chet Baker singing classics. Something in the slurry voice of that drug-addled trumpet player was especially soothing. Just as Baker had his career as a musician sidelined by heroin, Alan was being sidelined by his intermittent seizures.

By this time Alan was no longer my patient. Following my surgery, he was placed under the care of a neurologist, and my only communications would be one-sentence memos about the results of his scheduled MRI scans to ensure the tumour had not reappeared.

Alan's seizures continued but gradually abated in both frequency and intensity. He was able to return to that rustic Galiano cabin, this time on his own, intent on writing a new book.

Eventually, at the ten-year mark, I had one brief conversation with Alan on the telephone, confirming that he would not need any further MRIs. It was at this juncture that he mentioned some informal Sunday morning soccer games for men roughly in our age group at Trafalgar School, a tradition that had been happening for thirty years. I was curious. For decades, I had been too busy with work to consider organized sports. Alan assured me the vibe was gentlemanly, so I assumed it would be more leisurely than competitive.

It had never occurred to me that someone like Alan would go back to playing intense, full-contact soccer. As we've seen, the brain is normally surrounded by, and floats in, water (cerebrospinal fluid), and my surgery had disrupted that natural protective mechanism. The scarring that follows surgery may not allow the water to protect the brain in the same way. Any sudden head movements may therefore be more likely to result in harmful movements of the brain. The dampening hydrodynamic effects of the water could be lost.

I had never really thought much about what my patients ended up doing. It was the job of the neurologist to advise against risky activities; I was just the surgeon. My purview was the technical aspects of the physical problem, not the patient's lifestyle.

If Alan had asked me, I would have told him, "Soccer is very unpredictable. You cannot afford a concussion or any head injury." My nature would be to avoid any problems, and Alan's was to ignore the risks.

The doctor-patient relationship is unusual because it is mostly one-way. The patient tells you their most intimate fears and weaknesses, and you tell them what to do. You have a fiduciary responsibility to guard their secrets and act in their best interests, but they don't learn much at all about you. The patient interview is not a relaxed exchange of information; it's an interrogation. The doctor tries to extract the history of an illness without the patient's own perceptions incorrectly clouding the truth. Then the operation is a physical assault, a disfiguration designed to correct an imperfection as the patient lies naked and unconscious on the table. A profound level of trust is required. The doctor-patient relationship is designed to be unbalanced and finite. Generally I find it unsettling to bump into a former patient. They usually recognize me, and I stumble to remember who they are.

In 2011, ten years after I had removed Alan's brain tumour, I turned fifty. I had done some marathons and a few triathlons, but I had not participated in any organized sports since diving at the 1988 Olympics and had not played on a soccer team since I was a teenager. I decided to take up his invitation to check out that Sunday morning kick-around at Trafalgar Park. Long-distance running had become boring, and I craved the camaraderie of a team sport.

I was a striker—the one up front who tries to score. My strength was that I was faster than most. Like running from a lion, you don't have to outrun it, you just have to be faster than the guy beside you. What I gained in speed, though, I lost in ball control. My strategy was kick and run, not dribble. The long ball up the middle and the quick break. Not the beautiful game, but sometimes effective.

To my surprise, Alan stood out as the most vocal and intense of the competitors, and he headed the ball more than any other player. I would soon learn it was far more fun to play with him than against him. He would send long kicks up the field, and I would run on to the ball and try to score. I met another player, nicknamed DG, who had played semi-pro for Montreal Manic. David George was a very smooth player, pure finesse, a soccer artist. The three of us took special pleasure in combining with one another.

I never heard anyone mention the fact that Alan had had brain surgery. Perhaps nobody knew. As it did not seem to be a subject deemed worthy of conversation, I opted not to bring it up either. Certainly Alan didn't bring it up with me. Alan's personality was engaging—he conversed like a storyteller, joked with a sharp wit. I realized I had known him only as an anatomical problem to be solved, not as a human being. If you could be old friends in a moment, Alan engendered that feeling. I left that day feeling that this soccer thing would be better than I thought.

That is how I joined Alan's team, the Point Grey Pirates, in the fall of 2011. In the winter and spring, we practised Tuesday nights from 9 to 11 p.m. at the Point Grey turf and played games on Sunday mornings against teams throughout the Lower Mainland. We had some pretty good players, and the games were often feisty and intense. Gradually we developed that alchemy known as team chemistry.

Two years later, in the summer of 2013, several of us had an opportunity to join a Canadian team competing in the Over-50 soccer division at the World Masters Games in Turin—the world's largest multi-sport event. The first such games had been held in Toronto in 1985, and it had become a quadrennial event for athletes over thirty-five years of age. The Sydney World Masters Games in 2009 attracted 28,000 competitors, more than double the number of competitors in the 2000 Sydney Olympics.

Eight Pirates joined the squad—known as Vancouver United—that was going to Italy. Alan did not pass the strict medical tests required by the games organizers because of some heart issues. But a physician, who shall remain nameless, signed his consent form and the paperwork was duly registered.

We arrived in Turin during the scorching Italian summer heat. There were ten teams in our division; we were physically the smallest, but probably the fastest and fittest.

We won our first match, and in our second match the following evening against Australia, we won again, 3–0, but Pat, our star midfielder, was elbowed viciously in the throat. Pat himself was a physician and, sensing the injury could be serious, he slept that night on a sofa at an apartment that DG and Alan shared so he'd have company. The next morning, I took Pat to the best hospital in Turin to see an ENT specialist, who looked down his throat with a laryngoscope and quite literally said, *"Mamma mia!"* He motioned for me to look down the scope as well, and I saw a red swollen hematoma closing more than half of Pat's larynx. I asked him if he thought Pat might need a tracheostomy if things got worse. "Probably not." That afternoon I bought a Swiss Army knife and visited the Shroud of Turin in case either would be needed. Pat was out for the rest of the tournament.

Losing Pat, our star player, forced us to come together and play better without him. Each evening, I would rendezvous for pasta and Barolo with DG and Alan, and we would analyze the games loosely, with mutual admiration and hyperbole proportional to the number of bottles consumed. I felt twenty-six again. It was the same feeling as when I competed in the Seoul Olympics—only with wine and money. As we moved through the tournament, it felt like we were part of something special. I enjoyed the camaraderie with Alan and the team, and I felt more carefree than I could remember. My athletics had always been intensely competitive. As a diver, completing a three-and-a-half somersault was not enough; it had to be done better. Finishing an Ironman was not enough; it had to be done faster. This was different. This was pure joy.

Alan wrote up amusing game reports after each win, a purposeful exercise in building team morale. In the playoffs, it soon became apparent that because of our cohesiveness and teamwork, the team called Vancouver United was the team to beat.

We arrived at the finals—which would be played in the evening under floodlights, to avoid the heat of the sun—undefeated, and were disappointed to discover our opponents were not Italians or Brazilians or Germans, but rather a bunch of guys from Edmonton, Alberta. We prevailed 2–0. There was a rather moving rendition of "O Canada" during the medal ceremony, with everyone in the grandstand joining in. I had scored the most goals in the tournament and Alan had captained the defence, which allowed only two shots and one goal in seven games. Alan and I hoisted the trophy together.

We stood side by side under the floodlights on the warm Italian evening, surrounded by cheering, and paused for a picture.

———

To say that my inclination to be a brain surgeon in grade six was fortuitous is an understatement. I have been lucky to have access to education and the guidance of a series of mentors, and I know not everyone gets that opportunity. There might well have been a child in grade six on that soccer field in Liberia who was smarter than I was but destined for drudgery because of poverty and circumstance. Maybe the country's medical system will be able to support a neurosurgeon in the future and they will be the first. If that happens, I would tell that child, you will never be bored. The brain will impress you with its anatomical beauty and fascinate you with its functional complexity. On rare occasions, if you are listening, it will give up a secret about why it malfunctions, but it will withhold so many more. I would tell them, "Keep going, you have chosen the right path."

This book highlights just seven of the several thousand patients I have treated and benefited from knowing. Saika, the remarkable nine-month-old boy in Liberia who suffered with such a quiet dignity, taught me that we can fail as physicians, but we must always try to help. Jeff, whom I was lucky enough to meet when I was adrift in medicine with no clear focus, crystallized my decision to study surgery. Emily and Leo forced me to think beyond what I had been taught in medical school or what was known in my field. They encouraged me to treat an unknown condition and emboldened me to imagine there must be an Armando in the world with yet another unknown disease. Nadia humbled me—quite simply, neurosurgeons do not know everything about the brain, and there are some things in medicine that can only be explained as a miracle. Alan taught me to celebrate the life of a patient, which can be far more rewarding than defeating their illness. The real victories in medicine are macroscopic, not microscopic.

After a hundred years of neurosurgery, we have an excellent under-standing of the structure of the brain but remain ignorant about most of its higher functions. We can speak eloquently about its anatomy but lack an understanding of how thoughts are formed. We benefit from its creativity, imagination and logic but cannot explain how any of these processes occur. The brain's abilities are so complex they appear to transcend its physical form.

Many have suggested that the mind (thinking) and the body (brain) are separate. This mind-body dualism was formalized by René Descartes (1596–1650) in his *Meditations on First Philosophy*, in which he said the mind could exist without the body. His philosophy advanced the science of his day because physicians were then allowed to begin dissecting cadavers, since the soul was free to enter heaven without an intact body. I would argue, however, that this separation of mind from body is artificial and fundamentally wrong.

We can detect the footprints of thoughts—brain activity—with a variety of instruments. Severely brain-injured patients have no such activity. I am painfully reminded of this every time I have to speak with the parents of a young victim suffering head trauma from a motor vehicle accident. That is a tortured conversation, infinitely more difficult for the parents than for me, but nonetheless emotionally wrenching, even from across the room.

The brain thinks and because of these thoughts, we know we are alive. Descartes's famous "I think, therefore I am" summarized this reality. Several hundred years later, we still do not know how these thoughts are formed or created. The human brain, the most complex object in our universe, may one day be able to understand itself.

Although the understanding of how we think may still be a long way off, the understanding of how we feel may be closer at hand. This is a field I am increasingly drawn to—I believe it is the next frontier of neuroscience and that neurosurgery will play a pivotal role. Emotions can be triggered by the activity of certain brain regions. Electrical activity in the amygdala (an almond-shaped structure deep in the temporal lobe) is felt as intense fear. If an electrode is surgically placed in a patient's amygdala, to detect the origin of their seizures, for example, a tiny electrical current applied to that electrode will instantly trigger fear. The fear is intense and very real, complete with sweating and a racing heart. Fear is not an abstract concept; it is activation of your amygdala.

Similarly, a sense of euphoria can be triggered inadvertently when deep brain stimulation electrodes, inserted for Parkinson's disease, activate the deeper limbic pathway instead of the intended, more superficial, motor pathway. Patients feel euphoric and become disinhibited, then begin to behave inappropriately. One of my patients came into my office the day after their DBS was activated and kissed me. It was immediately obvious to me that something was wrong, but they were completely unaware. They returned to normal as soon as we adjusted the stimulation.

I am particularly interested in the pathway for sadness. Overactivity in this pathway and the resultant depression is alarmingly common in our society. It drives suicide and is a major factor in drug addiction. Our team has been treating severely depressed patients with brain surgery for the last twenty years. Chronically ill and refractory to all medical therapies, these patients present with the most devastating symptom—lost hope. We have documented that surgically disrupting this overactive pathway can lead to remarkable recoveries. We are just submitting our new theories on the pathway of depression to peer-reviewed medical journals for the experts in the field to judge. My hope is that this breakthrough in the understanding of depression will lead to new methods to alleviate it.

Medical exploration needs to continue to enable such break-throughs. As surgeons, we tend to optimize our time for the treatment of today's patients without thinking about those we cannot help. We avoid the difficult, the undiagnosed and the untreatable because they slow us down and steal precious time away from those more easily treated. The business of medicine does not remunerate pondering.

In 1990 a gynecologist from Indiana, Dr. Frank Meshberger, published an article in the *Journal of the American Medical Association* that made an extraordinary observation about Michelangelo's *Creation of Adam*, the famous painting that adorns the ceiling of the Sistine Chapel (and the one that my patient had thought about after a DBS operation stopped his tremor). Meshberger described the outline behind God as a perfect representation of the midline of the human brain. Anatomists around the world were dumbfounded by the obvious portrait of the inside of the brain that had remained unrecognized since 1512. Cadaveric dissection was rare in sixteenth-century Rome, but Michelangelo was known to "flay dead bodies in order to discover the secrets of anatomy." Da Vinci was also making the first drawings of the insides of the brain at that time. Michelangelo's painting had been thought for centuries to represent that moment from Genesis 1:27 when "God created man in his own image," but perhaps there was a deeper meaning. Michelangelo may have discovered the internal anatomy of the brain and wanted to show it and suggest that God's gift to Adam (who is clearly already alive in the painting) was not the spark of life but rather the gift of knowledge.

Medical learning and discovery is not just a science—it's also an art. Science teaches us how to study the problem, but there is an art to listening, to understanding the patient and to imagining the answer. Imagination and a sense of wonder are key ingredients in the path towards understanding. Just as important is the tenacity of the long-suffering patient, whose mysterious complaints are too often dismissed or misheard. After twenty-five years as a neurosurgeon, I have learned that listening to the most challenging patients can teach you the most profound truths. Truths about medicine, truths about yourself.

ACKNOWLEDGEMENTS

First and foremost, I would like to thank my wonderful patients—some given amusing pseudonyms in these stories, but most unnamed. I am indebted to all of them. They have allowed me the privilege of trying to help them, and in the process, I have learned about medicine and myself.

I was blessed with an excellent education, beginning in 6th Avenue Belleville in St. Michael, Barbados, and continuing to a trinity of Trinities: Trinity College School in Port Hope, Trinity College at the University of Toronto, and Trinity College at the University of Oxford. I am grateful to the University of Toronto's Faculty of Medicine and the University of British Columbia, where I did my neurosurgical training. I met my surgical mentor and fellow Caribbean, Dr. Felix Durity, in Vancouver, and he encouraged me to subspecialize and pursue my passion. Thank you also to Harvard University for teaching me surgical leadership skills.

Writing is a solitary pursuit that has many challenges, from thought to word to book. I would like to thank my editor, Amanda Betts, who has read and reread this manuscript and helped get what I was thinking down on paper. This book would not have seen the light of day without my agent, John Pearce. It is a pleasure to hear his voice and words of encouragement on the phone.

I am forever grateful to my family, who have always understood and respected this work that I do, where I am often responding to emergencies at inopportune times, day or night. Without their support I could never have dedicated the time required to discover these new diseases. Without them, I would never have met my "magnificent seven."

Finally, I would like to thank you, the reader, for taking this leap of faith with me on my first book. I hope this journey continues, as I have enjoyed writing this book and I hope you have enjoyed reading it.

NOTES

CHAPTER 4

A 2018 study in World Neurosurgery . . . David S. Kushner, John W. Verano, and Anne R. Titelbaum, "Trepanation Procedures/ Outcomes: Comparison of Prehistoric Peru with Other Ancient, Medieval, and American Civil War Cranial Surgery," *World Neurosurgery* 114 (June 2018): 245–51, doi: 10.1016/j.wneu.2018.03.143.

CHAPTER 8

I submitted the revised manuscript . . . and the paper was accepted May 13, 2016. Christopher R. Honey, Peter Gooderham, Murray Morrison, and Zurab Ivanishvili, "Episodic Hemilaryngopharyngeal Spasm (HELPS) Syndrome: Case Report of a Surgically Treatable Novel Neuropathy," *Journal of Neurosurgery* 126, no. 5 (May 2017): 1445–746, Epub July 8, 2016, doi: 10.3171/2016.5.JNS16308.

CHAPTER 10

We published the case report, and VANCOUVER syndrome entered the medical world . . . Christopher R. Honey, Marie T. Krüger, Murray D. Morrison, Baljinder S. Dhaliwal, and Amanda Hu, "Vagus Associated Neurogenic Cough Occurring Due to Unilateral Vascular Encroachment of Its Root: A Case Report and Proof of Concept of VANCOUVER Syndrome," *Annals of Otology,*

Rhinology & Laryngology 129, no. 5 (May 2020): 523–27, Epub December 1, 2019, doi: 10.1177/0003489419892287.

CHAPTER 11

In 2021, we submitted a medical paper using a new DBS that could steer the current precisely into "Nadia's target" . . . Krüger MT, Avecillas-Chasin JM, Heran MKS, Naseri Y, Sandhu MK, Polyhronopoulos NE, Sarai N, Honey CR, "Directional Deep Brain Stimulation Can Target the Thalamic 'Sweet Spot' for Improving Neuropathic Dental Pain," *Operative Neurosurgery* (May 2021), doi: 10.1093/ons/opab136.

CHAPTER 12

In 1990 a gynecologist from Indiana, Dr. Frank Meshberger, published an article . . . Frank Lynn Meshberger, "An Interpretation of Michelangelo's Creation of Adam Based on Neuroanatomy," *Journal of the American Medical Association* 264, no. 14 (Oct. 1990): 1837–41, doi: 10.1001/jama.1990.03450140059034.

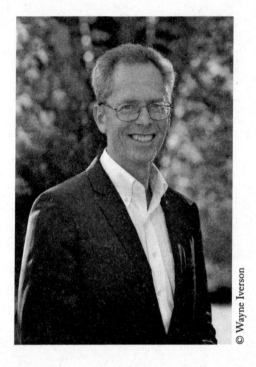

© Wayne Iverson

DR. CHRIS HONEY is a neurosurgeon at Vancouver General Hospital and Head of the Division of Neurosurgery at the University of British Columbia. He obtained his medical degree from the University of Toronto and his doctoral degree from the University of Oxford as a Canadian Rhodes Scholar. Dr. Honey lives in Vancouver with his family.

DrChrisHoney.com